X665
How Q
(Con)

COMPLEMENTARY AND ALTERNATIVE MEDICINES: KNOWLEDGE IN PRACTICE

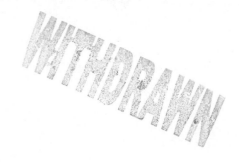
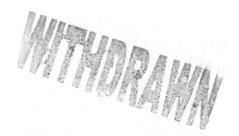
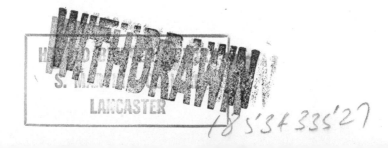
185343335'27

COMPLEMENTARY AND ALTERNATIVE MEDICINES

KNOWLEDGE IN PRACTICE

Edited by

SARAH CANT and URSULA SHARMA

FREE ASSOCIATION BOOKS / LONDON / NEW YORK

Published in 1996 by
FREE ASSOCIATION BOOKS LTD
57 Warren Street, London W1P 5PA and
70 Washington Square South, New York, NY 10012–1091

ISBN   1 85343 351 9 hardback
       1 85343 352 7 paperback

A CIP catalogue record for this book is available from the British Library.

Printing history: 99   98   97   96   4   3   2   1

Produced for Free Association Books Ltd by
Chase Production Services, Chadlington, OX7 3LN
Printed in the EC by J. W. Arrowsmith Ltd, Bristol

Contents

Notes on Contributors

Espen Braathen is an anthropologist employed as a special consultant at the Central Norwegian Competence Centre for Substance Abuse in Aalesund, Norway. His research interests include anthropological studies of alternative therapies and the new public health, socio-cultural aspects of and perspectives on psychiatric treatment and drug addiction, and the sociology of sports.

Helen Busby is Research Fellow at the National Primary Care Research and Development Centre at Salford University. She undertook her research training on medical (social) anthropology at Brunel University, where she developed a collaborative project with London Lighthouse about the use of complementary therapies by people with HIV and Aids (with Ian Robinson). Her research interests include people's knowledge and choices about both official and non-official forms of health-care.

Sarah Cant is Senior Lecturer in Sociology at the Roehampton Institute, London. She has written extensively in the areas of medical sociology and health policy, her most recent book being *Going Private: Why People Pay for Health Care* (1993). Her current research interests include the study of complementary medicine and social change.

Helle Johannessen is Magister and PhD in anthropology from the University of Copenhagen. Since 1983 she has been co-ordinator of the International Network for Research on Alternative Therapies, based at the University of Copenhagen. She is Research Associate at Slagelse National Institute for Social Educators.

Richenda Power has been in practice as a naturopath and an osteopath since 1983, working in the private and the public sectors, and in urban and rural settings. She conducted sociological research for her PhD (1991) on the emergence of 'holistic' medicine in Britain. Other responsibilities include being a tutor/counsellor for the Open University Social Science foundation course; external examiner for the General Council and Register of Osteopaths (UK), and module co-ordinator of 'Osteopathy and Society' for the MSc Osteopathy, European School of Osteopathic Medicine, UK.

Mike Saks is Professor and Head of the School of Health and Community Studies at De Montfort University, Leicester. He has been engaged in research into the relationship between orthodox and unorthodox medicine for a number of years. Aside from many contributions to conferences, journal and texts in this area, he is the author of *Alternative Medicine in Britain, Professions and the Public Interest: Medical Power, Altruism and Alternative Medicine*, and co-author of *Health Professions and the State in Europe* (with Terry Johnson and Gerry Larkin).

Ursula Sharma is a social scientist trained in both sociology and social anthropology. Her most recent work has been in the field of medical anthropology and she is the author of *Complementary Medicine Today: Practitioners and Patients*. She is employed as Professor in Sociology at the University of Derby.

Midge Whitelegg is Lecturer in Health Studies at the University of Central Lancashire, teaching the BSc course 'Health Sciences for Complementary Medicine'. She completed her PhD on 'Paradigm shifts and the use of science in orthodox and alternative medicine' at the School of Independent Studies at the University of Lancaster in 1994. She qualified as a herbalist with the National Institute of Medical Herbalists in 1988 and practises in a multidisciplinary clinic in Lancaster. She is currently Vice-president and Director of Research for the National Institute of Medical Herbalists.

Introduction

Sarah Cant and Ursula Sharma

Complementary medicines have proliferated dramatically in the United Kingdom (and indeed in other European countries) since the 1970s; the increase in number of practitioners (Fulder and Munro 1982) being matched by an increase in usage by consumers (MORI 1989). They are no longer marginal to the total system of health care (hence the label 'complementary' – though some still prefer to call them 'alternative' and the latter term is more commonly used in the United States). They therefore deserve our critical and reflexive attention. Their progress from a marginalized position to one of practical importance in most Western societies and many societies of the former Soviet bloc, has been marked by debates about the validity and role of their knowledge, their relationship to the established modes of medical knowledge and the reasons for their attraction to consumers. The purpose of this volume is to throw light on these issues in a way that will be illuminating both to social scientists and to those involved in the field of healing and medicine themselves.

Background to the Volume

In spite of the heated debates about the scientificity or otherwise of complementary medicines – which would suggest a polar opposition between orthodox and 'complementary' medicine – defining the field is not easy. We deliberately refer to 'medicines' in the title of this book to stress their great diversity. Some of the more established therapies, such as osteopathy, require their students to learn some elements of biomedical[1] knowledge. On the other hand, practices such as dowsing and some forms of 'New Age' healing are unlikely to gain medical recognition in the near future and are based on premises radically different from those which underlie biomedicine. Until very recently all the therapies popularly identified as 'alternative' or complementary' were in the same legal boat in Britain[2] (permitted to practise but not officially recognized by the state) and consequently practitioners have often been able to unite around various political issues. Yet there is a sense in which every healing mode has its own history and characteristics. Therefore any generalizations we make must be very cautious ones and charting a single unilinear account of the role and future of complementary medical knowledge is impossible.

If the diversity of complementary therapies is a problem for those who would attempt to understand their resurgence in general terms, the very boundaries between orthodox and unorthodox medicine are just as problematic. For many purposes it is quite legitimate to characterize orthodox biomedicine as an integrated system of knowledge based on a medical scientific view of the body (see Lock and Gordon 1988). On the other hand not all the therapeutic practices accepted by doctors in the biomedical clinic are actually based on or compatible with such knowledge. The medical profession is a broad church; a growing number of doctors are actually offering complementary therapies in some form (Anderson and Anderson 1987). An important section of the biomedical community aspires to some kind of holism, often identified as a distinguishing characteristic of complementary medicines. Mike Saks's chapter in this volume demonstrates that the boundaries between orthodox and complementary medicines are far from fixed.

Despite these complexities and caveats, we think that it is possible to consider the general significance of complementary medical knowledges within the context of wider theoretical debates about the nature of knowledge in contemporary societies. Why (and how) are some forms of knowledge accorded public legitimacy whilst others are discredited? What is the nature of expertise and how far does it disempower the non-expert? Is it true that modern societies are no longer held together by common forms of knowledge and values?

These are questions of political as well as theoretical importance, to which social scientists might be expected to contribute. Yet (with some interesting exceptions) medical sociologists and anthropologists have largely failed to bring complementary medicine within their critical gaze, being more occupied with the disjunctions between lay understandings of health and illness and those of the biomedical clinic. They have generally treated other healing modes with sympathy but as inhabitants of cultural sidelines and traditional backwaters (Sharma 1993; Cant and Sharma 1994b). These positions require re-evaluation in the light of the growth of this area of health care.[3] This volume is primarily an attempt to contribute to such a project by discovering how far recent ideas about knowledge deployed in the social sciences help us to understand the growth of complementary medicines, especially the social dynamics of the construction of their knowledge bases, their transmission, codification and ownership.

What happens, then, when we pull the complementary medicines in from the margins and give them centre stage? First, stepping out of the biomedical clinic and into the complementary practitioner's consulting room, removed from general debates about the relative merits of different forms of healing, it is possible to describe aspects of complementary medicine hitherto neglected. Complementary medical knowledge operates on a number of levels (formal and informal, local and general), be it the communication between practitioners, the activities of professional associations and the legitimation strategies employed, the use of the knowledge by patients or the encoding and decoding of the knowledge in practice. Knowledge is always 'knowledge in practice' and sociologists and anthropologists have established a fine tradition of empirical studies of biomedical 'knowledge in practice' (Atkinson 1988; Lock and Gordon 1988). If we focus on complementary medicines, we must not make the mistake of looking only at their codified and abstract forms.

Second, by bringing complementary medicines in from the margins we should be able to consider the development of these knowledges in the light of general theories about the role of knowledge in present and future societies. Do complementary medicines signify the collapse of the 'metanarrative' (Lyotard 1986) of science? Does the popularity of health care approaches that are not directly aligned to the traditional scientific paradigm suggest that science has lost its legitimating function? If so, how else is this knowledge of health and illness legitimated in the wider social arena? Are complementary therapists simply another kind of expert in a society that relies more and more on generalizable expert knowledge? Or, to the extent that knowledge is exchanged and shared among patients and practitioners of complementary medicines more than is the case in biomedicine, does this question the very distinction sociologists have made between lay and expert medical knowledge? These are all questions which lead us to engage with major debates about the role of knowledge in society.

In the remainder of this introduction we will discuss a number of theoretical ideas and positions that may help us comprehend the significance of complementary medical knowledges. The contributors to this book vary in the extent to which they engage with such theoretical perspectives explicitly, but they are offered to the reader to contextualize the contributions. We start by setting out some influential ideas about the role of knowledge in contemporary societies in general, then proceed to look at some of the concepts which have informed debates about the nature of medical knowledge in particular. Moving from these grander theories to the micro-level we consider the nature of local knowledge and conclude by considering how the insights gained from micro-studies of the complementary healing clinic, the healer and the patient might inform broader theorizing about knowledge.

The Significance and Role of Expert Knowledge in Advanced Industrial Societies: Implications for Complementary Medical Knowledges

No society can operate without knowledge, but it is the codification and specialization of knowledge that is significant in 'modern' societies. Expert knowledge has become a fundamental resource of social life (Bell 1973), so much so that commentators have described contemporary society as a 'knowledge society' (Stehr 1994). Giddens (1991) has similarly drawn attention to the centrality of 'expert systems', codified and generally applicable bodies of knowledge deployed and interpreted by experts, technicians and professionals and not accessible to the lay public. The development of expert knowledge, Giddens argues, is a product of the ever more complex division of labour and the increasing reliance on technology, but also the decreasing importance of local context, the disembedding of social relations and the 'tremendous acceleration in time–space distanciation which modernity produces' (Giddens 1991: 18), so much so that social life has to be organized around abstract systems, systems of activity and knowledge with a global currency. Social life is thus dominated by bodies of knowledge which are highly complex and increasingly distinct from 'lay' knowledge. In as much as they are codified these knowledge systems can be conceived as independent of the practitioners (whether lawyers, doctors, car mechanics or complementary practitioners), but practitioners/experts are still required to apply the knowledge systems for those people who do not have access to it. This knowledge may be scientific or technological, but equally it may concern social relations: 'The doctor, the counsellor and the therapist are as central to expert systems of modernity as are the scientist, technician or engineer' (Giddens 1991:18).

The pervasion of and reliance upon 'expert systems' in all areas of social life has led to the 'de-skilling' of those individuals without access to the knowledge and a devaluation of 'lay' and 'local' knowledge. Indeed it is the notion of professional knowledge which itself creates a category of 'lay' or 'local' knowledge, the other side of the 'expert' coin. Where knowledge of health and illness is concerned such lay knowledge has by no means disappeared; indeed we know that individuals engage in much self-prescribing and domestic care before seeking professional or expert help (Wadsworth *et al.* 1973). Yet even such popular knowledge is increasingly mediated to the lay public via experts, for example with the publication of books about folk remedies.

Let us explore further the ways in which expert knowledge is associated with power and the implications this has for the non-expert. As Rueschmeyer says of experts:

They define the situation of the untutored, they suggest priorities, they shape people's outlook on their life, they establish standards of judgement in different areas of expertise – in matters of health and illness. (Rueschmeyer 1986: 104)

In other words the expert, by virtue of his or her knowledge, can dictate to the non-expert appropriate ways of behaviour and living. Bauman shows us how expert knowledge, in the Enlightenment view of the relationship between knowledge and society, was conceived as having the power to be legislative, that is, it had a moral power that could not be explained purely in terms of its practical 'scarcity' value:

the authority involved the right to command the rules the social world would obey, and it was legitimated in terms of a better judgement, a superior knowledge guaranteed by the proper method of its production. (Bauman 1992: 11)

The tradition of healing which has come to be thought of as 'orthodox' medicine claimed (and was accorded) this legislative role in the course of the nineteenth century, gaining the logic and status to discredit other approaches as inappropriate, naive, even 'quackery'. It established its own knowledge as the only valid arbiter of acceptable medical practice and was granted moral powers that extended beyond its practical application. Complementary therapists today operate from a position of needing to establish their own credentials as 'experts' and their own worthiness of such moral legitimacy.

But where did orthodox medicine's powerful position come

from, and how was the medical profession able to legislate about what types of medical teaching could or could not be taken seriously? The sociology of the professions offers us important insights, examining as it does the processes by which occupational groups in general gain legitimacy and status as 'experts' in particular socially valued fields.

The Sociology of the Professions and the Legitimation of Knowledge

Early work on the sociology of the professions emphasized the possession of particular traits and attributes, such as membership of a professional association, a codified knowledge base (usually scientifically validated), altruistic values, and so on (Greenwood 1957; Goode 1960) to explain the high status and authority of professionals. More recent work has not denied the importance of such traits, but has given greater emphasis to the strategies actively deployed over time to engender such a position, such as social closure (Parkin 1974), state support (Johnson 1972; Larson 1977), market control (Freidson 1970; Larson 1977) and technical authority (Freidson 1970) and sees these as methods of securing autonomy of practice and a monopoly of provision. According to this framework, the possession of specialized/expert knowledge is still crucial (Larson 1977) since as well as legitimating high status it actually provides the means to activate social closure strategies (Freidson 1970). After all, if knowledge is deemed to be expert, only a small number of people with the appropriate qualifications and abilities will be in a position to mediate that knowledge.

Larson (1977) established that such knowledge would have key characteristics: it would be taught in an organized way, most usually in a university (or at least an institution that collects, transmits and eventually produces knowledge); and it would be standardized and accredited and often have scientific anchorage. The authority acquired by this kind of knowledge has served to shape the form and expectations of other knowledges. Thus, the standards set by orthodox medical knowledge – the long training, the limitation of the number of practitioners, the codification and standardization of medical education – have established important benchmarks against which to judge complementary medical knowledges. Expert knowledge gives some the privilege to speak, to act as arbiters.

It is also true that considerable collective and political organization on the part of an occupational group is required to generate and maintain knowledge of this order; the sociology of the professions is very largely the study of the politics of knowledge. Larkin's (1983) concept of 'occupational imperialism', for instance, shows how the medical profession was able to control the market by subordinating other groups in the medical division of labour as technical aides (for example, physiotherapists), or allowing them either a 'separate but contained' status (for example, opticians) or a 'separate but low' status (for example, chiropodists became professionals supplementary to medicine). Wardwell (1962) employs a similar approach when he classifies health occupations in the medical division of labour. For example, 'limited practitioners' are those whose health services are focused on particular parts of the body – for example, dentists. 'Ancillary' professions are those which are dependent on medical supervision, for example, nurses.

The knowledge imparted in the training of members of these subordinate groups was defined as ultimately dependent upon the principles laid down by biomedical authority, although recently some groups, notably nurses and midwives, have attempted to re-define their knowledge bases in their own terms. Establishing that the orthodox medical knowledge base was indeed 'expert' knowledge was in itself only part of the process of gaining legitimacy and authority. The professional project in addition involved the framing of the position and status of other groups in terms of the priority claimed for the knowledge base of orthodox medicine.

Notwithstanding what we said earlier about rescuing complementary medical knowledge from the margins, both Larkin's and Wardwell's approaches suggest that we cannot disregard the *relation* of any healing profession to the medical profession, or the relation of their knowledge to the biomedical knowledge base. The situation, however, has never been static. In the nineteenth century the orthodox medical profession was only able to banish homoeopathy to a marginal status with some struggle (Nicholls 1988). Saks's chapter in this volume shows how the medical profession was able to dismiss other forms of medical care as quackery yet eventually incorporated selected aspects of acupuncture knowledge and practice when it became untenable and foolhardy to discredit this approach. The medical profession has not acted uniformly in relation to other knowledge systems but the concept of occupational imperialism is still useful, provided that we do not uncritically assume that the patterns of domination of the past will also be the patterns of the future.

In fact medical attitudes towards complementary medicines have changed dramatically within the past ten years. The 1986 BMA report on alternative therapies was highly dismissive of the knowledge claims of complementary medicines as unscientific and of most of their treatments as unproven. Yet it evidently did not convince the public, and a subsequent report published in 1993 took a completely different tack. Complementary medicine now attracts vocal lay and tacit governmental support and is not so easy to dismiss. Thus, whilst the medical profession may still try to subordinate or appropriate complementary medicines, the practitioners are less likely to lie back and accept what is delivered to them. At the same time there is evidence that orthodox medicine may itself be subject to forces of deprofessionalization, that is, its own power and authority is open to change as a product of economic forces (McKinlay and Arches 1985) and a reduction in the knowledge gap between doctors and their patients (Haug 1973). The growing popularity of the 'subordinate' group and the diminishing power of the 'dominant' group may provide for a more level playing field and may well account for the institutional rapprochement between orthodox and some complementary therapies.

The ascendance and power of scientific orthodox medical knowledge does not mean that 'non-scientific' forms of knowledge have been eradicated – this book is testimony to a contrary reading. Nevertheless, those complementary medicines which have succeeded in obtaining the right to state registration in Britain (to date osteopathy and chiropractic) are those which have also managed to convince the medical profession that their knowledge is not incompatible with medical science (Cant and Sharma 1994a). It seems apposite then to explore the continued pervasiveness of the scientific paradigm, the reasons for the high status it has been accorded and the extent to which complementary practitioners are persuaded of its value.

The Social Construction of Knowledge:
Science as a Special Case

Conformity to scientificity was a shibboleth imposed by the medical profession as a condition first of recognizing other healing groups at all, then later, as positions softened, for recognizing them as partners of some kind within the NHS. Why has science (not just medical science) been accorded such legitimacy in the first place? Partly, no doubt, because the claims of objectivity and value freedom have served to place 'science' at the top of a hierarchy of knowledge, so much so that sociologists of knowledge at one time declared scientific knowledge beyond the scope of social, political, cultural and economic analyses (Merton 1973).

Since the 1960s sociologists have argued that such a reading is inadequate and that scientific and medical knowledge are as much a product of social and cultural processes as lay and non-scientific knowledge. The work of Kuhn (1970) was path-breaking in this regard. In particular the concept of the paradigm has in itself 'revolutionized' our thinking about knowledge. Kuhn established that science is characterized by phases of very conservative practice followed by periods of revolutionary upheaval. Scientists, he suggested, are not (as they see themselves and claim to be) totally open-minded enquirers, but approach the exploration of the world from vested theoretical positions – they operate within a paradigm, a whole way of thinking and working which filters what they are likely to find acceptable or unacceptable in new work or in other traditions. The enduring value of the Kuhnian approach for an understanding of the contemporary experience of complementary medical knowledge is demonstrated by Whitelegg who offers a compelling account of the way in which medical science rejected the herbalists' method of analysing the comfrey herb (Whitelegg, this volume). Protagonists of complementary therapies themselves have deployed Kuhn's analysis to argue that the ridicule directed at them by medical scientists is derived from the incompatibility of their ideas with the orthodox paradigm (Graham 1990: 232; MacEoin 1990). Nevertheless, Sharma's contribution suggests that some complementary groups try to accommodate scientific knowledge on their own terms, establishing connections with bodies of scientific knowledge which are not necessarily those which the medical profession demands, and creating their own interpretations of scientific theories. Cant's chapter suggests that engagement with the scientific paradigm is still a prerequisite when groups of practitioners desire legitimacy and that at this juncture the engagement may not be on their own terms at all.

Kuhnian analysis, however, treats the production of scientific knowledge as a relatively self-contained domain. Sociologists such as Barnes (1985) went further and established the influence of social, political and economic interests on the shaping of knowledge. Saks (this volume) details how such interests have operated in the experience of complementary medicine in general and Cant's study of homoeopathy and chiropractic documents how these two groups have transformed their knowledge in response to changing demands from the state and medical profession. Without these pressures it is not clear whether changes to the knowledge base would have occurred and this points to the importance of contextualizing the alterations to complementary medical knowledges.

Kuhn remains important since he has been influential with complementary medical practitioners who see his relativization of orthodox scientific knowledge as potentially liberating, as speaking to their condition, but also because the strength of the scientific paradigm is not to be underestimated. Practitioners have also appealed to writers such as Feyerabend and Capra (for example, Graham 1990) to support the argument that the rejection of complementary medical knowledges is a product of a limitation on the part of scientists themselves with respect to their own science, blinkered to the implications of newer ways of doing science or to the need for a plurality of ways of generating knowledge. Complementary medical knowledge can then be seen as avant garde rather than antiquated.

In summary, science has occupied a position of high status but it has taken a major shift within the sociology of science to recognize the social, cultural and economic factors which shape scientific knowledge. Such a recognition, however, also alerts us to the need to subject complementary medical knowledges to a similar analysis.

The Social Role of Knowledge: Power and Control

In the end we cannot study science as a self-contained institution. It is essential to study it in terms of its relationship to powerful groups outside the academy and research laboratory. Various social science perspectives have effectively questioned the very separability of science from power, or of knowledge of nature from political process (Latour 1993).

In relation to medicine and healing this integration of knowledge and practice has largely been discussed in terms of the ways in which medical knowledge relates to social control. The empirical relationship between medical ideas and social control is well rehearsed (Szasz 1971) and sociologists have illustrated how medical knowledge has transformed its form and function as a means of regulating the patient and providing the practitioner with status (Jewson 1976). However, the theorist who has had the most pervasive influence in recent studies of medicine and healing is Foucault (1975). Foucault does not treat knowledge as a separate domain located in some kind of history of ideas; knowledge is located in discourse. Medicine is a discursive practice, a way of carving up the world, looking at it and talking about it; moreover one of relatively recent origin (though other discourses about the body and healing went before). He describes how, in the eighteenth century, the practice of medicine more and more involved the objectification of the patient, the by-passing of the patient's reported experience of his or her symptoms, in favour of the subjection of the body to the penetrating 'gaze' of (increasingly scientific) medical enquiry – which in this century quite literally penetrates the body with scanning devices of various kinds. The rise of a medical practice based on this objectifying 'gaze' is related to the requirement for more precise modes of surveillance and control of populations (Foucault 1975; 1977). However, the exercise of the medical gaze is not simply 'influenced by' or 'a product of' the needs of the state or any other agency. *Chez* Foucault, the exercise of the medical gaze *is* the exercise of power itself, for power is dispersed and embedded in practices – the practices of the clinic as much as the practices of the state bureaucracy, the penitentiary, the militia, the police, even the family.

Knowledge, then, is a much more concrete thing than the term 'discourse' might imply. Some medical sociologists who have tried to apply Foucauldian ideas have tended to treat medical knowledge as primarily manifested in discourses, understood as mainly lin-guistic practices, albeit having consequences for bodies, overlooking this incorporated nature of knowledge itself (for example, Lupton 1995: 156). In *The Birth of the Clinic* (Foucault 1975: 120) there is a passage where Foucault comes close to identifying medical knowledge as what Mauss called a 'technique of the body', a socially learnt way of using the body, albeit experienced as entirely 'natural' by those who practise (Mauss 1973). In this context the 'gaze' can also be seen as what Bourdieu (1986) has termed 'habit-us', a learnt disposition of body/mind/emotion. Foucault also fore-shadows the anthropologists who have developed the idea of embodiment (Csordas 1994; see also Busby, this volume) by repre-senting knowledge as a matter of 'concrete sensibility', as the very term 'gaze' suggests.

Where does all this leave complementary medicine? We could conceive of complementary medical practice as a site of what Foucault calls 'resistance'. This is a rather undifferentiated concept for Foucault but a very necessary one, for power invariably engenders resistance of various kinds – resistance is even described as the 'com-patriot' of power (Foucault 1980: 42). Certainly many users and practitioners would regard complementary medical practice as repre-senting a positive protest against certain aspects of biomedical knowl-edge and practice.

Or we could, as some critics have suggested, see the rise of complementary medicines as signifying simply a different way of practising power. Thus the principles of holistic medicine can be deployed in occupational health care programmes to facilitate greater productivity and compliance, as Kotarba has suggested in relation to programmes designed for the care of US astronauts (Kotarba 1983). Espen Braathen's chapter argues (in relation to homoeopathy) that it is not even a question of whether the individual is controlled more effectively by complementary medical institutions, but of how complementary medicines assist (through their stress on individual responsibility for health) the effecting of *self*-discipline, the creation of the disciplined bodies (and minds) which, as Foucault has shown, becomes more and more of a necessity for the body politic.

Complementary medicines have the capacity to be involved simultaneously in medicalization and demedicalization processes (Lowenberg and Davis 1994), both the increase and decrease of dependence on therapeutic experts. Social scientists who have studied complementary medicines have tended to focus on the liberating role of complementary medicine. For example, Busby's contribution describes how Chi Kung allows the patient the opportunity to know their own bodies and enhance self-awareness and understanding. But an alternative reading, in terms of complementary medicine's capacity to effect a self-responsible but politically conformist subject, is always possible.

Local Knowledge and the Clinic

Foucault and those who have worked in his tradition undermine claims that real medical knowledge, the most valuable, is created primarily by the medical scientist in the laboratory, though medical science may of course be considered an important form of discourse among others in the realm of health care. Medical knowledge is above all created and reproduced in the clinic. Foucault has not been the only theorist to note this. There is a long tradition of empirical micro-studies in medical sociology and anthropology which make the same point. For example, Atkinson (1988) studied the construction of medical knowledge in the interaction between tutors and students on the hospital ward and showed that some important concepts and practices are not learnt primarily from the codified knowledge in textbooks but through the observation of the particular teacher at work, at the patient's bedside. Much medical education is experiential and uncodified, consisting of the acquisition of certain dispositions, as Lella and Pawluch's (1988) account of students dissecting a cadaver shows. Good has shown how medical schools cultivate a certain kind of moral subjectivity in students, for example, through learning to write up a case, to look for signs and symptoms, to 'think anatomically' about people. Pedagogical and clinical practices reproduce forms of knowledge parallel to the kind which appears in examination papers; implicit, unformulated but crucial for professional practice (Good 1994: 65ff). Thus even orthodox medical knowledge has a large component which is tacit and non-standardized. It is a matter of regret to us that this volume does not include any comparable study of complementary medical training institutions. However, Power's chapter illustrates the ways in which naturopathic knowledge is produced not just in the naturopathic academy but in the clinic, by the individual practitioner 'herself. Let us consider further what the study of the complementary clinic can tell us about the ways in which knowledge is engendered and maintained.

Biomedical knowledge in its abstract form is presented as the scientific and generalizable knowledge of every-body and no-body, which may obscure the fact that it is nonetheless *socially* produced and reproduced. Complementary practitioners also acquire generalizable knowledge of how sickness is caused and cured, how bodies work with minds, and so on, from their training schools, but to the extent that they subscribe to a holistic notion of health which stresses the particularity of the individual patient, they may expect to deal more with individuality than typicality in their everyday clinical practice. Moreover they require and usually develop (see Sharma 1995) a 'local' knowledge of how the kinds of patients they treat tend to behave, of which other complementary practitioners in the district are competent enough to warrant patient referrals, and of which neighbourhood GPs are sympathetic and which not. The practitioner acquires a bank of local data about his or her particular clientele in the form of notes on their diagnoses, schematic diagrams of their bodies, and so on, and, as Power's chapter shows, this information also becomes a resource for the practitioner, possibly a source of further generalizable knowledge. Johannessen's chapter shows that the practitioners' knowledge may be local in another sense – they develop localized versions of whatever therapies they have learnt, applying them in individualized, even idiosyncratic forms.

Local knowledge is of course a somewhat heterogeneous and clumsy term, which has been used to cover all those diverse kinds of knowledge which are not covered by concepts like 'expert system', which do not claim universality, or to be 'placeless principles' (Geertz 1983: 218). We use it here to include the tacit knowledge (Wainwright 1994: 150) involved in craft or other skills, knowledge based on personal experience, forms of knowledge which may be relatively explicit, even codified, but do not claim universal application (such as many forms of traditional healing), knowledge about localities, and so on. A major problem is that 'local', as a concept, is always in danger of becoming a subordinate or residual term, created by an analytic privileging of abstract systems over tacit knowledge, of 'global' cultural forms over those of the periphery (Wolff 1991: 166) (rather in the way that the concept of resistance becomes a residual term consequent upon Foucault's privileging of power). In the therapeutic context 'local' knowledge can cover most of the transformations which the knowledge of an individual patient's body might undergo before it is fed into the expert system delivered by the academy. Conversely, the term 'clinical experience' is a coded way of referring to the accumulation of local knowledge of particular bodies, and in some therapies the relatively small number of practitioners with long experience has caused problems in providing the necessary supervised clinical practice for the new wave of students in the academy.

The very slippery quality of local knowledge raises the question of who actually owns such knowledge? The knowledge incorporated into expert systems is managed by the institutions which confer the relevant kind of accreditation. It does not belong to these institutions as such; indeed their credibility rests on the claim that the knowledge they reproduce is universal, that (unlike commercial knowledge) it does not belong to individual persons or corporations even if they have the capacity to control its supply. However the ownership of knowledge is perhaps more controversial than this characterization would suggest. There is, as Harrison (1995) has pointed out, much cultural diversity (and sometimes ambiguity) with respect to the ground rules according to which the ownership and circulation of knowledge is managed. Some indigenous peoples have no doubt lost out when the dispersed local ethno-scientific knowledge of the healing properties of forest flora is appropriated by multinational pharmaceutical companies. When an important piece of genetic engineering is accomplished using DNA derived from tissue taken from a medical patient, does that innovation in no way 'belong' to the human being which has provided the necessary genetic material?

More relevant to our present context is the apparently mundane issue of the ownership of patients' notes. These are effectively an inscribed knowledge which mediates between the concrete local knowledge of the individual patient's body as comprehended by the physician, and the abstract system of therapeutic knowledge. This issue is now regarded as fairly well resolved in the NHS, at least as far as patients' access to notes is concerned, but as Power's chapter points out, it is far from clear in the field of complementary medicine. At what point in the transformation of local knowledge can practitioners be said to 'own' knowledge of the patient's body, to acquire the right to transform this knowledge into some other more general kind of knowledge, to use it for their own research ends?

Perhaps the most local form of local knowledge is the knowledge which the patient has of his or her *own* body. It has often been noted that biomedicine tends to discount such knowledge in favour of abstract and 'objective' knowledge of the body (Taussig 1980), whilst complementary practitioners, like traditional healers in many parts of the world, are more likely to regard the patient's own knowledge of his/her body, symptoms and circumstances as the very starting point for diagnosis and treatment. If practitioners claim to treat individual patients rather than disease categories (as in homoeopathy), then it cannot be otherwise.

Looking at the situation from the point of view of the patient, the transaction of knowledge is a two-way process. Not only does the patient deliver knowledge of his/her body, emotions, circumstances, and so on, to the practitioner, but the practitioner delivers knowledge about the therapy to the patient. The extent to which the process of therapy is conceived as an educative process varies from therapy to therapy and practitioner to practitioner, but the idea that treatment should be a learning process is widespread (see Sharma 1995). Anthropologists have repeatedly suggested that if therapy is efficacious, its success largely derives from its very capacity to effect a shift (through symbolic or other means) in the way the patient understands and evaluates his or her own symptoms (for example, Dow 1986). Busby's chapter shows how engagement with a Chinese form of therapy did not so much transform individuals' knowledge of their own bodies, but provided a new context for recognition of experiences, one which legitimated their experience rather than (as biomedicine had) invalidated it. Johannessen makes a similar point when she describes how various kinds of therapists structure the patient's experience of his/her body and health condition. In any case, the patients/clients make what they will of the complementary therapist's 'expert' knowledge and the outcome may actually be seen as a product of the interaction of their respective knowledges.

We are thus faced with an interesting contradiction. On the one hand, expert knowledge and abstract systems are more important than ever before. On the other hand, not all knowledge is located with the expert; indeed complementary medicines suggest the possibility of a re-skilling of 'lay' individuals, in as much as most of them involve some conscious attempt to re-educate the patient or help him/her to develop more self-understanding. Medical knowledge (and this is true of biomedical as well as complementary medicines) is, therefore, in the forms in which we actually encounter it today, at the same time disembedded and embedded, local and global, general and contextual, abstract and embodied. Hence the subtitle of this book – 'Knowledge in Practice'.

The Future of Knowledge

Great debate has raged about the future of knowledge. The postmodernists have vociferously argued that the failure of science to maintain general social assent to its claims to universal authority on the basis of its objectivity has opened the way to a plurality of knowledge claims, a situation in which many knowledges coexist without any one subsuming the others. In these terms, the emergence of 'complementary' therapies could be seen as evidence of the eventual collapse of orthodox medicine's epistemological authority. Lyotard (1986), for example, has argued that the postmodern age is characterized by 'an incredulity towards the metanarrative'. The 'Enlightenment project' adhered to the notion of scientific knowledge as rational, progressive, universal, true, objective and superior. It was 'legitimated' politically and gained social authority by recourse to a set of 'stories' which referred to ideas such as progress, the ever increasing control of nature, 'the dialectics of the spirit, the hermeneutics of meaning, the emancipation of the rational or working subject, or the creation of wealth' (Lyotard 1986: xxiii). Lyotard is rather vague about why the metanarrative which legitimates science as the supreme form of knowledge loses authority, although he talks about the increasing computerization of society and the 'mercantilism of knowledge' with associated prerequisites for efficiency and the increasing realization (already foreshadowed in the scientific project itself) that it is impossible ever to have absolute knowledge. The metanarrative and in particular the authority of science is thus replaced by knowledge that has validity by virtue of its performance. The vacuum left by science, he argues, is filled by numerous discourses/language games which are all capable of generating their own authority, none having privileged status. Other writers, coming to the problem from a variety of different political and intellectual experiences, identify postmodernity as a state of culture, emergent or yet to come, in which fragmentation is experienced not necessarily in negative terms of dissolution and disintegration but in terms of re-enchantment, enriching diversity and choice.

Bauman suggests that the fall of the legislative power of knowledge in a changing world (1992), 'the demise of the power-assisted universals and absolutes' (Bauman 1995: 6), is characterized primarily by uncertainty and is a feature of postmodernity. We can certainly apply such a reading to medicine. Where orthodox medicine used to legislate against inappropriate or naive beliefs by eradicating what it saw as erratic, barbaric or exotic medical practices, it can no longer fulfil this role as its own knowledge is open to question. This thesis has implications for the role of the professional/expert. If the experts' knowledge is no longer legitimated by the notion that the specialized knowledge they control is different from other forms of knowledge because it is objective, universal and rational, must they not suffer a loss of prestige and esteem? Bauman indeed suggests that intellectuals have had to shift from being legislators to interpreters of many sets of knowledge claims, no longer the purveyors of a single unitary truth. Thus the orthodox medical profession, it seems, is abandoning the simple discrediting of alternatives on the grounds of their unscientificity (the approach it took in the first BMA report on alternative therapies published in 1986) in favour of the role of the disinterested but experienced guide to patients in their choice of therapies. Its second report on complementary therapies (BMA 1993) stresses 'good practice' rather than scientificity, and calls for orthodox medical practitioners to delegate care to other therapists (who must be able to exhibit their competence) whilst retaining overall responsibility for the patient. It even suggests that orthodox doctors could provide the complementary therapies themselves.

For Lyotard, the postmodern demise of the legitimating metanarrative sees a fragmentation of knowledge into micronarratives which rely more on performativity (it does not matter about the theoretical basis but only whether knowledge 'works'), a highly empirical judgement. The reality of such performativity is difficult to discern. On the one hand the philosophical foundations of some complementary medicines can only with great difficulty be made to conform to the scientific metanarrative of orthodox medicine (Cant, this volume) and practitioners may prefer to gain legitimacy from endorsement by patients. It is also true that both complementary and biomedical procedures are increasingly subject to audit rather than scientific trial; the question that is being asked is not 'Is the knowledge on which these procedures are founded objectively correct?' but 'Do these procedures/interventions deliver the results which they are supposed to deliver?' In biomedicine the emphasis on performativity takes also takes the form of the introduction of streamlined management and performance indicators (Strong and Robinson 1990).

The criterion of performativity certainly permits a plural approach to health care and creates space for a heterogeneous set of knowledge claims which, for some members of the public (and a growing number), have equal validity. That is, each micronarrative is directed to a particular audience and has its own forms of validation, and biomedicine certainly seems to have lost its universal epistemological authority.

On the other hand, there is evidence to suggest the continued importance of a metanarrative, and a desire on the part of the practitioners to know more than just that their practice 'works'. Sharma's chapter shows that homoeopaths do search for means to legitimate their practical knowledge by grounding it in wider cultural concepts, some scientific and some not. Similarly Cant (this volume) argues that in the public arena the legitimating function of science still holds good and that in many complementary medicines there has been an engagement with the paradigm of orthodox medicine and an acceptance of many orthodox biomedical principles. Lyotard's observations would seem to be premature rather than incorrect where complementary medicines are concerned.

Rather than a rejection of the metanarrative, then, there appears to have been a merging and intertwining of different narratives which do not necessarily operate independently or have equal status. For instance, the development within the medical profession of groups of doctors who have wanted to adopt a more holistic approach (evidenced, for example, by the inauguration of the British Holistic Medical Association in 1986), could be seen as an expansion of the orthodox paradigm to rescue its pervasiveness in a changing medical context (and to claw back the patients?). Yet biomedical holism does necessitate a revision of the triumphalist metanarrative of scientific biomedicine, a recognition of the limitations of the Cartesian model on which the latter is based. In practice it is associated with a practical acceptance that some complementary approaches have a worthiness, even if the biomedical holists still believe that doctors should retain responsibility for the patient and delegate care.

The shift to performativity does raise interesting questions about the future of various medical knowledges in the light of the realization that expert knowledge may deliver problems as well as benefits. If the application of expert knowledge delivers the greenhouse effect, increasing environmental degradation, iatrogenic disease, and so on, then the very knowledge that sustains society is uncertain (Beck 1992). The rise of knowledge generally has been declared to have a dark side; it does not simply provide acceptable responses to the dilemmas of the social world but may generate unintended and unacceptable consequences (Giddens 1990; Beck 1992).

This leaves us with another contradiction. At the beginning of this chapter we cited Giddens's (1991) concept of the dependence of modern society on experts and their knowledge. And Stehr reminds us that 'everyone must still defer and under some circumstances is forced to defer to the authority of experts today' (Stehr 1994: xv). On the other hand, in spite of the emphasis on performativity, this expert knowledge does not necessarily deliver the goods and non-experts may become more discerning, reflexive and questioning of their dependence upon these systems. We come full circle to the opportunities for re-skilling by the non-expert.

To overcome this paradox, Giddens (1991) isolates the importance of relations of trust; users of the knowledge must be able to trust that providers and mediators of the knowledge will indeed offer them the best information. Knowledge is not legitimated purely in terms of either epistemological foundation or performativity, but in terms of its capacity to generate stakeholders' trust in the experts' integrity. Cant argues in her chapter that the professional project of complementary medicines has been directed, in part at least, to the acquisition of this trust through the assertion that their knowledge bases are safe and watertight and their professional competence guaranteed.

Our analysis of the material presented in this book, in the light of the recent literature on the sociology of knowledge, suggests that where medicine is concerned, Lyotard's characterization was premature, rather than incorrect. We do not find (as yet?) a total collapse of metanarratives nor that medical knowledge is acceptable only in terms of its performativity, for it is difficult to argue that legitimation simply descends to the level of practice and the wholesale acceptance of local knowledges. Knowledge may have become more plural but still has to justify its credibility and validity.

Concluding Remarks

Recent studies in the sociology and anthropology of knowledge have tended to emphasize the linkages between what sociologists used to call the micro and macro levels of analysis. But the more general theorizing work has tended to privilege the macro, concentrating on achieving some kind of general characterization of the kind of society that is emerging, and how it is different from that which has gone before. These are valid questions, but in answering them the insights derived from studies of specific occupational groups and their workplaces, of the ways in which their knowledge is communicated among themselves and others, of the ways in which 'lay' people use and make sense of expert knowledge, sometimes seem to get lost.

We think that the study of complementary medicines as represented by the contributions in this volume throws important light on the ways in which knowledge is transformed, both through explicitly political and through informal local processes. The contributions collected here also tell us much about the ways in which diversity is engendered and managed. They tell us a lot about continuity and discontinuity. The history of complementary medicine is discontinuous in that the emergence of a dominant medical orthodoxy pushed it into a particular position and the current revival is only partly a simple revival of something that went before, for complementary medical knowledge has been transformed. On the other hand, whatever sociologists like to think about so-called 'traditional' societies, and in spite of attempts to equate plurality with postmodernity, there is no doubt that therapeutic diversity at the local level is nothing unusual. It is probably characteristic of any society above a minimal level of scale and complexity that healing practices are diverse and may even rest on fairly diverse sets of assumptions about the body and the way it can be healed, even if these are not well articulated or legitimated in the public or official spheres. Self-healing and complementary medical practices are not completely new phenomena, but they had, until recently, escaped the control of legitimating authorities linked to the state or powerful elites and had not come to the attention of the funding authorities because of their very locality, their invisibility, the camouflage of implicit knowledge. Under these conditions, even when they have come to the notice of interested elite groups, the latter may not have the means to eliminate them. The novel factor in the post-1970s situation was not the existence of diverse healing modes in itself but the enormous boost in their popularity among consumers, a question that still needs to be explored more thoroughly.

In the West the modern emergence of biomedicine as having power to confer legitimacy did bring these local healing practices under scrutiny and in time led to their marginalization. Some have re-emerged, often in new forms and joined by recent inventions or importations from other cultures, to challenge this authority. We are far from seeing a delegitimated postmodern profusion, rather a period of intense contestation in which hybrid forms and strategic realignments will emerge. This might eventually lead to such de-centred postmodernist profusion, or (just as likely) to new modes of legitimation.

We hope that this introductory discussion has served to intro-duce the reader to a number of theoretical debates and questions that are apposite for an understanding of complementary medical knowledges. We hope that we have done this in a way that is intelligible and useful both to readers with a background in the social sciences and to those whose primary interest is in the thera-pies themselves. The remainder of this edited collection is divided into sections, each preceded by a brief introduction. Notwithstand-ing contributors' diversity of approach, we also draw some tentative conclusions at the end of the book, where some of the themes touched upon here will re-emerge.

Notes

1. Biomedical knowledge refers here to orthodox understandings of the pathology and physiology of the human body as taught in medical schools.
2. The majority of the contributions to this volume refer to British mate-rial. However, despite legal differences and some variation in the range of therapies that are regarded as 'complementary', there are many parallels between the situation in Britain and that in most European countries, in the US and in the mainly white/Anglophone 'Old Com-monwealth' countries. Therefore we feel that our discussion in this introduction has very wide applicability.
3. It is estimated that there are currently 160 therapies on offer in the UK, that between one in four and one in seven people have consulted a practitioner (*Which?* magazine, October 1987; November 1992) and that the number of training colleges and therapists has escalated (Cant and Sharma 1994b).

References

Anderson, E. and Anderson, P. (1987) 'General Practitioners and Alternative Medicine'. *Journal of the Royal College of Practitioners* 37: 52–5.

Atkinson, P. (1988) 'Discourse, Descriptions and Diagnoses: Reproducing Normal Medicine', in M. Lock and D. Gordon (eds) *Biomedicine Examined*. Dordrecht: Kluwer Academic Publishers.

Barnes, B. (1985) *Interests and the Growth of Knowledge*. London: Routledge.

Bauman, Z. (1992) *Intimations of Postmodernity*. London: Routledge.

Bauman, Z. (1995) *Life in Fragments. Essays in Postmodern Morality*. Oxford: Blackwell.

Beck, U. (1992) *Risk Society. Towards a New Modernity*. London: Sage.

Bell, D. (1973) *The Coming of Post-Industrial Society*. New York: Basic Books.

BMA (1986) *Alternative Therapy. Report of the Board of Science and Education*. London: BMA.

BMA (1993) *Complementary Medicine: New Approaches to Good Practice*. London: BMA.

Bourdieu, P. (1986) *Distinction: A Social Critique of Judgements of Taste*. London: Routledge and Kegan Paul.

Cant, S. and Sharma, U. (1994a) *Professionalisation in Complementary Medicine*. Final Report to the Economic and Social Research Council.

Cant, S. and Sharma, U. (1994b) 'Social Aspects of Complementary Medicine'. *Medical Sociology News* 19(3): 25–7.

Csordas, T. (ed.) (1994) *Embodiment and Experience. The Existential Ground of Culture and Self*. Cambridge: Cambridge University Press.

Dow, J. (1986) 'Universal Aspects of Symbolic Healing: A Theoretical Synthesis'. *American Anthropologist* 88: 56–69.

Foucault, M. (1975) *The Birth of the Clinic: An Archaeology of Medical Perception*. New York: Vintage Books.

Foucault, M. (1977) *Madness and Civilisation: A History of Insanity in the Age of Reason*. New York: Vintage Books.

Foucault, M. (1980) *Power/Knowledge. Selected Interviews and Other Writings 1972–1977*. Brighton: Harvester Press.

Freidson, E. (1970) *Profession of Medicine: A Study of the Sociology of Applied Knowledge*. New York: Harper and Row.

Fulder, S. and Munro, R. (1982) *The Status of Complementary Medicine in the United Kingdom*. London: Threshold Foundation.

Geertz, C. (1983) *Local Knowledge. Further Essays in Interpretive Anthropology*. New York: Basic Books.

Giddens, A. (1990) *The Consequences of Modernity*. Oxford: Polity Press.

Giddens, A. (1991) *Modernity and Self Identity*. Oxford: Polity Press.

Good, B. (1994) *Medicine, Rationality and Experience. An Anthropological Perspective*. Cambridge: Cambridge University Press.

Goode, W. (1960) 'Encroachment, Charlatanism and the Emerging Profession: Psychiatry, Sociology and Medicine'. *American Sociological Review* 25: 902–14.

Graham, H. (1990) *Time, Energy and the Psychology of Healing*. London: Jessica Kingsley.

Greenwood, E. (1957) 'Attributes of a Profession'. *Social Work* 2: 44–55.

Harrison, S. (1995) 'Anthropological Perspectives on the Management of Knowledge'. *Anthropology Today* 11(5) (October): 10–14.

Haug, M. (1973) 'Deprofessionalisation: an alternative hypothesis for the future'. *Sociological Review Monograph* 20: 195–211.

Jewson, N. (1976) 'The Disappearance of the Sick Man from Medical Cosmology 1770–1870'. *Sociology* 10: 225–44.

Johnson, T. (1972) *Professions and Power*. London: Macmillan.

Kotarba, J. A. (1983) 'Social Control Function of Holistic Health Care in Bureaucratic Settings: The Case of Space Medicine'. *Journal of Health and Social Behaviour* 24: 275–88.

Kuhn, T. (1970) *The Structure of Scientific Revolutions*. Chicago: University of Chicago Press.

Latour, B. (1993) *We Have Never Been Modern*. Hemel Hempstead: Harvester Wheatsheaf.

Larkin, G. (1983) *Occupational Monopoly and Modern Medicine*. London: Tavistock.

Larson, M. (1977) *The Rise of Professionalism*. California: University of California Press.

Lella, J. and Pawluch, D. (1988) 'Medical Students and the Cadaver in Social and Cultural Context', in M. Lock and D. Gordon (eds.) *Biomedicine Examined*. Dordrecht: Kluwer Academic Publishers.

Lock, M. and Gordon, D. (eds) (1988) *Biomedicine Examined*. Dordrecht: Kluwer Academic Publishers.

Lowenberg, J. and Davis, F. (1994) 'Beyond Medicalisation and Demedicalisation: The Case of Holistic Health'. *Sociology of Health and Illness* 16(5): 579–99.

Lupton, D. (1995) *The Imperative of Health. Public Health and the Regulated Body*. London: Sage Publications.

Lyotard, J. (1986) *The Postmodern Condition: A Report on Knowledge*. Manchester: Manchester University Press.

Mauss, M. (1973) 'Techniques of the Body'. *Economy and Society* 2(1): 70–88.

MacEoin, D. (1990) 'The Myth of Clinical Trials'. *Journal of Alternative and Complementary Medicine* 8(8): 15–18.

McKinlay, J. and Arches, J. (1985) 'Towards the Proletarianisation of Physicians'. *International Journal of Health Services* 18: 191–205.

Merton, R. (1973) *The Sociology of Science: Theoretical and Empirical Investigations*. Chicago: University of Chicago Press.

MORI (Market and Opinion Research International) (1989) *Research on Alternative Medicine*. London: MORI.

Nicholls, P. (1988) *Homoeopathy and the Medical Profession.* London: Croom Helm.

Parkin, F. (1974) 'Strategies of Social Closure in Class Formation', in F. Parkin (ed.) *The Social Analysis of Class Structure,* London: Tavistock.

Rueschmeyer, D. (1986) *Power and the Division of Labour.* Cambridge: Polity Press.

Sharma, U. (1993) 'Contextualising Alternative Medicine. The Exotic, the Marginal and the Perfectly Mundane', *Anthropology Today* 9(3): 13–18.

Sharma, U. (1995) *Complementary Medicine Today. Practitioners and Patients* (revised edition). London: Routledge.

Stehr, N. (1994) *Knowledge Societies.* London: Sage.

Strong, P. and Robinson, J. (1990) *The NHS Under New Management.* Milton Keynes: Open University Press.

Szasz, T. S. (1971) *The Manufacture of Madness.* London: Routledge and Kegan Paul.

Taussig, M. (1980) 'Reification and the Consciousness of the Patient'. *Social Science and Medicine* 14B: 3–13.

Wadsworth, M. E. J., Butterfield, W. and Blaney, H. (1973) *Health and Illness: The Choice of Treatment.* London: Tavistock.

Wainwright, H. (1994) *Arguments for a New Left. Answering the Free Market Right.* Oxford: Blackwell

Wardwell, W. (1962) 'Limited, Marginal and Quasi Practitioners', in H. Freeman (ed.) *Handbook of Medical Sociology.* Englewood Cliffs, NJ: Prentice Hall.

Wolff, J. (1991) 'The Global and the Specific: Reconciling Conflicting Theories of Culture', in A. King (ed.) *Culture, Globalization and the World-System.* Basingstoke: Macmillan.

PART ONE

Legitimating Complementary Medical Knowledges: History, Strategies and Obstacles

It is possible to produce an account of the history of complementary medicines that suggests clear phases of collective growth, decline and revival. In the first place it can be argued that the plural medical market of the eighteenth century was replaced by the monopolistic rise of orthodox medicine and the concurrent discrediting of other forms of medical care as quackery. The re-emergence of other forms of medical practice in the 1960s and 1970s was perceived as threatening by orthodox practitioners and the response was to discredit them or at least to portray them as distinct and alternative to orthodox practice. Lately, it appears that orthodoxy has become more favourably disposed to some of these alternatives so much so that it is prepared to view them as complementary to orthodox medical care. However, this historical description does not entirely capture the specificity of experience for each individual complementary therapy group, the dynamics of the changes, nor the range of strategies that has been undertaken by complementary medical groups themselves in their attempts to establish greater public legitimacy. Nor does the emphasis upon the reactions of orthodox medicine, important as they are, sufficiently capture the importance of social, economic and political changes that have underpinned the changing experience of complementary medicines.

In this section, Mike Saks documents this general history and, through the example of acupuncture, illustrates the specific reactions of orthodox medicine. Sarah Cant recognizes the importance of the medical profession, but charts the recent changes that have taken place within homoeopathy and chiropractic and the internal strategies that have been undertaken by these professions to enhance the public legitimacy and trustworthiness of their knowledge and practice. The groups have engaged with the scientific paradigm and have modified some aspects of their official and codified knowledge bases accordingly, but in so doing have experienced many unforeseen and undesired consequences as well as greater public standing. Finally in this section, Midge Whitelegg gives a detailed case study of the attempts to discredit and ban the comfrey herb. Here she shows that legitimacy is not contested on a level playing field; the strength of the medical paradigm has served to blinker the legislators to the healing properties of the herb.

In all three chapters the importance of the social and political context in which knowledge is articulated and legitimated is established. The social authorization of knowledge is not in practice a matter of the perceived truth or falsity of the knowledge alone but is also determined by the power and strategies employed by a number of players. These include the medical profession, the general public and the government as well as the complementary medical groups themselves.

1 From Quackery to Complementary Medicine: The Shifting Boundaries Between Orthodox and Unorthodox Medical Knowledge

Mike Saks

Introduction

This chapter takes a historical overview of the development of health knowledge as applied to practice from the sixteenth century to the present day, focusing on the relationship between orthodox and unorthodox medicine in Britain. The driving force behind the development of health knowledge can be conceived in a number of ways at a macro-theoretical level, ranging from the class-based Marxist approach that emphasizes the formative influence of the relations of production under capitalism through to the more consensual functionalist model stressing the importance of the needs of the broader social system (Hart 1985). In this contribution, however, the market-based neo-Weberian approach is considered to be the most helpful theoretical framework for analysing the shifting boundaries between orthodox and unorthodox medical knowledge – centred as it is largely on the interest-based turf battles between leading elements of the medical profession and practitioners of alternative medicine within the wider socio-political context.

The concept of interests is variously defined in the literature, with a significant divergence between conceptualizations derived from subjectively expressed preferences as opposed to *a priori* theorizing. Such interests are seen in this chapter, though, as being advanced by actions that objectively enhance the position of the occupational groups concerned in relation to power, status and income – as determined by the balance of costs and benefits arising in any particular situation. In this frame of reference, competing interests are viewed by neo-Weberians as being linked to the legally underwritten, monopolistic position gained by professions in the marketplace. The British medical profession is regarded as illustrative of an occupation that has so effected social closure, by securing a privileged position in the health care market. From a neo-Weberian perspective, it is argued that, in the contest over the boundaries of orthodox and unorthodox medical knowledge, the medical establishment has generally managed successfully to defend its own professional interests in face of the challenge posed by outsiders. This in turn has fundamentally shaped the development of ideas and practice in the health arena, including their differential pattern of institutional legitimation (Saks 1995).

This does not mean, however, that there have been no changes over time in the nature of the knowledge underpinning the orthodox health care division of labour, nor that the interests of unorthodox therapists in gaining wider state-based legitimacy have been completely unrealized. In fact, as this chapter indicates, the dividing line between orthodox and unorthodox medical knowledge has shifted considerably of late, with new opportunities opening up for less conventional therapies to be practised under the umbrella of orthodoxy – even though the process of moving from being cast as 'quackery' to a position arguably more akin to 'complementary' medicine over the past two centuries has been far from straightforward. Such historical trends are considered in broad-brush terms, recognizing that there are variations in the position of specific therapies which cannot be explored fully in detail here.

Before proceeding further, it should be noted that the concept of unorthodox medicine at present covers a very wide range of therapies, from osteopathy and herbalism to homoeopathy and acupuncture. It must be stressed, though, that it is not the knowledge base itself which is the critical arbiter of whether a particular therapy is considered to be part of unorthodox medicine, but rather the extent to which it receives formal recognition from the state, with appropriate support from the medical profession. It is in this sense that the alternative medical knowledge of today can become the mainstream medicine of tomorrow. Despite greater degrees of medical recognition, however, therapies centred on this form of knowledge have still not been that widely supported institutionally – whether through systematic inclusion in the mainstream medical curriculum or the receipt of significant official research funding (Saks 1992).

This said, the main principles on which unorthodox health knowledge is rooted in the contemporary era do empirically tend to deviate from the 'scientific' biomedical model that currently underpins orthodox medicine, centred on the conception of the body as a symptom-bearing organism. Although some groups of alternative therapists have sought to forge a closer alliance with orthodox bodies of knowledge of late, they can still generally be viewed as being more holistically oriented, in so far as they bring together body, mind and spirit in diagnosis and treatment to a greater extent than is characteristic of conventional medicine (McKee 1988). Herein lies a major strand of the challenge which many unorthodox therapies have brought to orthodox medical knowledge since the professionalization of medicine in Britain from the mid-nineteenth century onwards. The evolving boundaries between orthodox and unorthodox medical knowledge thereafter can be highlighted with reference to the period of two or three centuries leading up to the first half of the nineteenth century. This throws into perspective the relativity of the current position, indicating that the clearer lines of separation between the orthodox and unorthodox which were to develop are themselves a novel phenomenon.

Early Patterns of Health Knowledge and Practice

In this earlier period, a relatively open market existed for the various forms of health care on offer, in which there was no national monopoly of the range of health knowledge underpinning such practices as the wearing of amulets to cure illness and the use of herbal remedies and charms to alleviate suffering (Larner 1992). It was not, therefore, easy to classify any particular group of health care practitioners as representing 'orthodoxy'. This has not, of course, stopped some commentators from illegitimately projecting the present back on the past and elevating surgeons, apothecaries and physicians to a position they did not attain until the mid-nineteenth century (Wright 1979). In reality, herbalists, bonesetters and the like competed with the occupational forerunners of the emergent medical profession at this time on a far more level playing field than today in a fee-for-service system in which it was impossible clearly to differentiate practitioners in relation to the length and content of their training or even the therapies employed (Porter 1989).

This is not to say, however, that an incipient, albeit much less powerful and smaller, regular medical community could not be identified, based on the establishment of the Royal College of Physicians and the licensing of surgeons and apothecaries from the sixteenth century onwards (Larner 1992). As Jewson (1976) indicates, in the seventeenth and eighteenth centuries 'bedside medicine' was to the fore in the practice of such groups, in which wealthy paying clients could influence the form of both diagnosis and treatment and there was a greater appreciation of the need to interpret illnesses on the basis of a wider conception of the individual. In this context – at a time when self-help was much more in vogue and the power of the developing profession over the medically unlicensed was very limited in a predominantly *laissez-faire* society (Porter 1987) – there was considerable overlap in the health knowledge employed by practitioners. It should not be surprising, therefore, that up to the eighteenth century senior figures in the prestigious Royal College of Physicians followed their competitors by engaging in such practices as astrology, which in Britain today would certainly be defined as being based on unorthodox knowledge (see Wright 1979).

In this period the concept of the 'quack' tended to be used by medical practitioners to vilify those outside their ranks who were seen to be practising medicine in bad faith, not least by operating without appropriate qualifications and depending mainly on the sale of unproven and often dangerous secret remedies (see, for example, Maple 1992). As Porter (1989: vii) notes, though, even here the boundaries between orthodox and unorthodox knowledge were still blurred and contested: 'Altruistic doctors did not confront thievish quacks like white meeting black ... Rather the panorama presents individual medical practitioners of many stripes, some more, some less, engaged in quackish activities.' Much the same could also be said of those who were not regular practitioners – ranging from those employing their remedies on a pragmatic, empirical basis to those with a more theoretically informed frame of reference – leaving a real sense of ambiguity about the basis of attribution of the term 'quackery' in the years leading up to the early nineteenth century (Porter 1994).

However, this ambiguity – in which the concept of 'quackery' was also applied to those with medical qualifications themselves – was to disappear with the formation of the modern medical profession, in which the designation of 'quack' became increasingly firmly associated with practitioners outside this more tightly delimited professional group. There were signs of the increased marginalization that this symbolic shift implied as early as the first half of the nineteenth century when the newly formed Provincial Medical and Surgical Association (the predecessor of the British Medical Association) began to flex its muscles as it lobbied for a medical register. This led to attacks on rival practitioners like homoeopaths and hydropaths from the 1830s onwards in both popular tracts and the medical journals, which depicted them as 'money grubs' generating a trail of 'carnage'. Whilst this assault was ideologically justified in terms of the desire 'to protect the public from those who defrauded, injured, or killed the sick' (Bartrip 1990:42), the potential gains from this strategy were great in terms of the self-interests of the elite and rank-and-file of the profession at a time when many of its members were financially hard pressed, not always of the highest status and in a less than secure political position to assert their monopolistic claims (Saks 1995).

The attempt officially to delineate the boundaries of a marginal sphere of the unorthodox by leading medical figures, however, was initially restricted by the fact that juries all too rarely supported prosecutions for violations of medical jurisdictions. This was understandable at a stage when there was large-scale popular support for the myriad of rival practitioners and tight internal control of the incipient profession could not be maintained because of the large number of licensing bodies and medical theories in existence (Porter 1987) – even though prestigious bodies like the Royal Colleges could still prevent those with undesirable therapeutic connections from taking up its training posts and force even quite eminent practitioners, like Professor John Elliotson, to resign their posts because of their link with marginal belief systems (Parssinen 1992). Much stronger efforts, however, were made to ensure that the emerging realm of unorthodox medical knowledge was formally sidelined as the mid-nineteenth century approached. This paralleled attempts by medical practitioners to present a more unified stance based on the development of 'scientific' medicine as they strove to depart from the health care pluralism of earlier times in Britain by gaining the legally underwritten standing of a fully fledged profession (Stacey 1988).

The Rise of the Medical Profession and the Development of Scientific Medicine

The more enforceable boundaries that resulted from the professionalization of medicine through the 1858 Medical Registration Act served as a basis for a state-legitimated assault on unorthodox medicine in all its forms. Such marginalized practices were henceforth even more firmly labelled as 'quackery', to the obvious detriment of their exponents. In this respect, it should be stressed that there would have been no distinctly ascertainable field of unorthodox knowledge had not the medical profession gained ascendancy in Britain through the legislation enacted from the mid-nineteenth century onwards. This gave the profession its monopolistic position in health care underpinned by the legally enshrined right, amongst other things, to the title of doctor, to engage in self-regulation, to sue for fees and to claim to treat certain categories of illness (Saks 1992).

With the establishment of the unified medical profession following the 1858 Act, the main threat to its position from the now more clearly defined realm of the unorthodox came from external rivals who were allowed to practise under the Common Law. This threat was amplified by practitioners who employed unorthodox therapies within the medical profession itself. In line with its own professional self-interests based on enhancing power, status and income, the medical response to alternative therapies followed a dual pattern during the ensuing century, encompassing both the regulation of deviant insiders and a continuing campaign against outsiders – who in turn strove to defend their market position by proclaiming the greater relative safety and efficacy of their remedies compared to orthodox medical practice (see, for example, Brown 1987). At the heart of the regulatory activity was a medical elite which included leading figures in the Royal Colleges and the British Medical Association. This elite, supported by the medical colleague network, employed a range of strategies in its response to the unorthodox, from negative ideological invective against its external competitors to the striking off of deviant insiders – in face of which rival practitioners were increasingly powerless as the latter half of the nineteenth century wore on (Saks 1995).

In the heightened attack on 'quackery' outside medicine that contributed significantly to the process of boundary definition, the medical elite capitalized on the common register and undergraduate medical curriculum which added greater coherence to the profession (Stacey 1992). It was thereby able to ensure that entrants to the profession were more focused around the evolving 'scientific' biomedical principles of first hospital and then laboratory medicine on which the new orthodox medical knowledge came to be based (Jewson 1976). 'Hospital medicine' took the classification of disease as the central point of the process rather than the individual, in contrast to the more holistic tendencies of herbalists and homoeopaths now operating at the margins of orthodox health care (Brown 1985; Nicholls 1988). This was later supplanted by 'laboratory medicine' in which the body was conceived as a complex of cells, with therapeutic intervention increasingly based on laboratory diagnosis. This emergent medical framework further increased the social distance between practitioner and patient as compared to many competing bodies of knowledge which, leaving aside much of nineteenth-century proprietary medicine that symbolically identified with orthodox medicine for commercial purposes, typically adopted a more personalized approach to treatment than allopathy (Brown 1987).

This developing edifice of 'scientific' medical ideas enabled the profession starkly to demarcate on its own terms the boundaries of orthodox and unorthodox knowledge. In this task, the fact that medical registration was required to sue for fees and be employed by the state played a critical role in legitimating medical orthodoxy in the latter half of the nineteenth century (Berlant 1975). The regulation of alternative medicine was further facilitated by the adoption by the General Medical Council of an ethical code that limited co-operation with unorthodox outsiders (Inglis 1980). In addition, a growing number of medically controlled journals – not least the *British Medical Journal* and the *Lancet* – criticized medically unqualified practitioners for being irrational and robbing patients of their money (Saks 1995). This attack by the orthodox medical journals was also aimed at deviant insiders who were said to undermine the dignity of the profession. The use of such invective was a potent deterrent to doctors given its adverse effects on career enhancement, as research increasingly became central to the generation of medical knowledge. Ostracism was often employed too by the colleague group to restrict medical interest in homoeopathy and other challenging forms of alternative therapy (Nicholls 1988).

The growing cohesion of the profession around the more clearly delineated boundaries of orthodox medicine following the 1858 Act undoubtedly strengthened its regulatory position, even if it did not mean that disputes between the Royal Colleges and the British Medical Association were totally laid to rest (Berlant 1975). From the standpoint of medical interests, the subsequent assault on unorthodox forms of medical knowledge could be explained in terms of the difficulties of gaining full professional standing, which materialized in medicine only after seventeen bills had been presented to Parliament in rapid succession (Waddington 1984). This meant that there could be no easing of effort if the monopolistic privileges of the profession were to be maintained and extended, especially given the challenge that the pragmatic empiricism and conflicting theories of healers, naturopaths and other unorthodox practitioners posed to the increasingly unified knowledge base of orthodox medicine. The structure of medical interests was also sharpened by the low income of most doctors compared to many alternative therapists, including the homoeopaths who thrived on an upper-class clientele of nobility and royalty (Nicholls 1988).

By the same token, the detrimental effects of the actions of the medical profession on the interests of alternative practitioners should not be ignored for, by the turn of the century, the number of such therapists had dwindled significantly (*Report as to the Practice of Medicine and Surgery by Unqualified Persons in the United Kingdom* 1910). This trend appears to have continued as this fragmented body of practitioners were also disadvantaged by the subsequent development of state medicine – particularly through the National Health Insurance Act of 1911 and the National Health Service Act of 1946 which gave doctors pre-eminence as suppliers of medical services in the vital state sector of the market (Berlant 1975). Although this did not stop groups like the herbalists and osteopaths from endeavouring unsuccessfully to encroach on such exclusive legal rights in the 1920s and 1930s, the medical establishment was the key player in determining the fundamental shape of the boundaries of orthodox health knowledge at this stage. In this role it was aided by a medical–Ministry alliance that was to ensure that the evolution of a succession of subordinated health care occupations including midwifery, nursing, physiotherapy and occupational therapy took place under the auspices of medical dominance (Larkin 1992; 1995).

The many benefits to medical interests of the close relationship of the medical profession to the state in the process of boundary setting were also apparent in the legislation passed in the 1930s and early 1940s restricting the claims that could be made by non-medical practitioners in the treatment of such conditions as cancer, diabetes and epilepsy (Vaughan 1959). In this light, alternative medicine clearly posed a reduced competitive threat to orthodox medical interests in the interwar years, especially since the medical elite still possessed powerful internal controls over medical careers in the first half of the twentieth century. This seems to have inhibited Sir Thomas Horder from further researching radiesthesia after his official enquiry into this subject and to have led to Axham being struck off the medical register for serving as an anaesthetist to Barker, the acclaimed bonesetter (Inglis 1980). Such controls were most potent, though, through the gatekeeping role of medical education, journals and research funding which kept unorthodox medical knowledge at the margins, even in the hands of qualified doctors (Saks 1995).

Pressure for changing the boundaries between orthodox and unorthodox medical knowledge, however, started to mount from the mid-twentieth century to the early 1970s as public interest in the alternatives began to increase. The by now consolidated professional domination of the state-financed health service, though, enabled the professional elite to inhibit the development of unorthodox medicine, despite the establishment of more rigorous programmes of training in areas like acupuncture and hypnotherapy (Fulder 1988). This was epitomized by the role that it played in this period in turning down applications from osteopaths and chiropractors to join the professions supplementary to medicine (Fulder and Monro 1981). Informal patterns of referral by doctors to unorthodox practitioners were also reduced by an escalating campaign to denigrate 'quackery' in the medical journals, at a time when co-operation was still formally prohibited and associations with alternative medical knowledge remained negatively regarded by the profession (Saks 1995).

However, the medical profession was not completely successful in limiting the practice of unorthodox medicine, as demonstrated by the inability of the British Medical Association in the 1950s and 1960s to prevent spiritual healers from gaining access to National Health Service hospitals (Inglis 1980). Generally, though, the tactics deployed were effective in defending established conceptions of orthodox and unorthodox medical knowledge. This is apparent from the way in which the medical elite used its capacity to determine the pattern of entry to its own ranks, the content of the undergraduate medical curriculum and the growing allocation of medical research funding, from which non-medical exponents of unconventional therapies were effectively excluded. At the same time, local medical committees commonly rejected proposals to study alternative therapies like traditional flower remedies (Eagle 1978), while unorthodox medicine carried such stigma in the profession that in the early 1970s medical members of the Scientific and Medical Network, an organization committed to the exploration of fringe knowledge, were unhappy about their identities being publicized (Inglis 1980).

The Modern Resurgence of Unorthodox Medicine

Such previously marginalized therapies as osteopathy and herbalism, though, underwent a resurgence from the mid-1970s onwards. This pointed the way towards a greater degree of complementarity in the relationship between orthodox and unorthodox medicine, inspired not only by the now substantial numbers of members of the public who avail themselves of the services of unconventional practitioners and use self-help remedies, but also by the enhanced support that such therapies have attracted in political circles in contemporary Britain (Saks 1994). These factors, together with the further development of the strategies of professionalization adopted by a number of groups of unconventional practitioners, have helped to prompt a reconsideration of the boundaries between orthodox and unorthodox medical knowledge, such that the medical profession in Britain has now taken steps to incorporate more reputable unconventional therapies like acupuncture into its own repertoire (Saks 1995). In this context, it is clear that the association of unorthodox medicine with 'quackery', which was so strongly historically forged in the wake of the professionalization of medicine, has finally begun to recede.

Having said this, the elite of the profession until very recently largely maintained its adversarial position against non-medical practitioners of unorthodox knowledge in defence of orthodox science. This is exemplified by the report of the British Medical Association (1986) on alternative therapy which extensively documents the triumphant march of medical science before assailing unorthodox medicine for being unscientific and linked to medieval superstition. None the less, a more incorporationist stance has now been increasingly taken by the medical profession, particularly by grassroots practitioners. This was initially prompted in the higher echelons of the profession by the decision of the General Medical Council in the mid-1970s to end its ethical prohibition on referrals from doctors to unorthodox therapists, as long as the doctor was in control of the treatment regime (Fulder and Monro 1981).

This decision helped to pave the way for growing numbers of doctors to apply unorthodox medical knowledge in their own practice either directly or through the professions allied to medicine with which they work – and more recently to subcontract such services within the new internal market in the National Health Service to the wide range of unorthodox therapists, from aromatherapists to chiropractors, now in private practice in Britain (Saks 1994). The direction of the shift in the boundaries of medical knowledge that this represents is illustrated by the transformation of the generally sceptical response of the medical profession to acupuncture in the early 1970s into a position whereby in the late 1980s small amounts of orthodox funding became available for research in this area, doctors increasingly employed acupuncture in their practice and more items were published on this subject in the mainstream medical journals. On a broader front, it has also more recently resulted in legislation which has given osteopaths the right, *inter alia*, to protection of title – if not the fully enfranchized standing of medicine within the state sector (Saks 1995).

In terms of interests, the elite of the medical profession could afford to continue to adopt a defensive stance in its reaction to unorthodox medical knowledge in the years immediately following the mid-twentieth century. This position, however, was less and less tenable from an interests' viewpoint as the second half of the twentieth century unfolded. With rapidly growing public demand for unorthodox therapies from the 1970s onwards, at a time when the counterproductive side-effects of modern medicine were becoming ever more apparent, orthodox knowledge came under increasing challenge (see, for instance, Pietroni 1991). This did not initially impinge on the state medical monopoly of practice, for there were still relatively small numbers of unconventional practitioners both inside and outside the profession. However, there was a growing threat of the medical profession losing patients in the private sector to such therapists and experiencing a reduction in its hard-won power and status. This helps to account for the more overt attack on unorthodox medicine that developed in this period, followed by the medical incorporation of the alternatives as the elite of the profession came under growing siege from within and without in the increasingly pluralist state political structure.

From this standpoint, the incorporationist strategy of the medical profession in which the boundaries between orthodox and unorthodox medical knowledge could be seen to be breaking down was further encouraged from the late 1970s onwards by the assault on the power base of the profession by successive Conservative governments, committed to fostering consumerism and opening up competition (Alaszewski 1995). This was complemented in the 1980s by the allocation of ministerial responsibility for alternative therapies and the establishment of the all-party Parliamentary Group for Alternative and Complementary Medicine. At the same time, the lobby for unorthodox medicine was strengthened further by rising consumer interest in including alternative medicine within the National Health Service (Saks 1992). This backcloth in large part explains the spiralling growth of the number of unorthodox therapists, which even by the early 1980s had reached over thirty thousand in more than fifty associations covering a fast expanding range of alternative therapies (Fulder 1988).

Although divisions within the ranks of alternative practitioners continue to exist, their own interest-based lobby has also been enhanced by the recent drawing together of many previously disparate elements in unorthodox medicine through such bodies as the Confederation of Healing Organizations and the Council for Acupuncture, as well as the establishment on a wider scale of organizations like the Institute for Complementary Medicine and the Council for Complementary and Alternative Medicine (Saks 1992). Given this mounting challenge, the incorporation of the alternatives by orthodox medicine – while keeping their non-medical exponents under fire or at least in a position subordinate to the profession – clearly enables the medical elite not only to rebut the challenge to its power, status and income, but also to create new empires to colonize in the public and private sector.

However, it is important to note that, in spite of this strategy, the shifts that have recently occurred in the boundaries between orthodox and unorthodox medical knowledge are limited. This is highlighted with reference to acupuncture, which has been incorporated into medicine in a selective manner as an analgesic on the basis of orthodox neurophysiological explanations, rather than as a broad-ranging practice centred on traditional Oriental philosophies (Saks 1995). This can clearly be interpreted as another means of constraining the internal and external development of unorthodox medicine in the interests of the medically qualified, by restricting the terms of incorporation. This case underlines the point that the redefinition of the dividing line between orthodoxy and unorthodoxy has usually been where the knowledge concerned is complementary to medicine, rather than in any sense conflictual.

The stretching of boundaries through incorporation has typically therefore not occurred where unorthodox therapies are based on radically different principles to orthodox biomedicine, with its underlying belief that the body is like a machine, the parts of which can be repaired on breakdown (McKee 1988). Despite changes within biomedicine itself in recent years that have enabled greater recognition to be given to the role of the mind in diagnosis and treatment, the whole person conception underlying many classic unorthodox therapies has generally not been encapsulated by the profession at a philosophical level (Lyng 1990). Nor have practitioners of such therapies necessarily been much enamoured with working with doctors and allied health professions outside of the independent sector because of the constraints that this imposes on practice (Sharma 1992). In the case of homoeopathy the additional overlay of the twin notions that like cures like and the more dilute a remedy the more effective it may be, have sat even less easily with medical orthodoxy, despite the handful of homoeopathic hospitals that have traditionally existed within the health service (Nicholls 1988).

The limits to the incorporation of unorthodox knowledge within medical orthodoxy are well illustrated by the latest publication of the British Medical Association (1993) on what is now viewed as 'complementary' medicine. The position it takes focuses more on the most appropriate method of regulating such therapies than condemning unorthodox medicine outright. This apparently more liberal stance, however, can also be seen as a means of ensuring that unconventional therapies remain within prevailing structures of professional dominance. This point is accentuated by the support that the British Medical Association gives to the delegation of tasks to non-medical practitioners, whilst upholding the principle of medical responsibility for the patient; the advocacy of the profession's own model for regulating the unorthodox, including codes of ethics and a core curriculum based on such medically oriented subjects as anatomy and physiology; and the persisting reliance on the arguably less than appropriate methodology of the randomized controlled trial for evaluating unorthodox health care knowledge at a time when insufficient medical resources are available for conducting large-scale trials in this area (Larkin and Saks 1994). Clearly, there are prices to be paid for the incorporation of unorthodox therapies into medical orthodoxy as 'complementary' medicine.

Conclusion

None the less, from the foregoing discussion it is clear that there have been considerable shifts in the boundaries between orthodox and unorthodox medical knowledge over time in Britain. In this sense, after the relatively open field which existed prior to the mid-nineteenth century was transcended, the marginal position of unorthodox medicine seems to have been slowly transformed in the contemporary era – to a point where it is on the verge of wider acceptance. This reflects general trends in both Europe and the US in which the popularity of unconventional medicine has also grown in recent years, paralleled by its increasing incorporation into medical orthodoxy (see Lewith and Aldridge 1991; Eisenberg *et al.* 1993, respectively). The broader international significance of this phenomenon raises important questions about whether a more integrated state-based health system will emerge in Britain in the future, especially given past tensions between unorthodox practitioners and leading figures in the medical profession.

Whatever the future form of health provision, however, this chapter has also shown that the shifting boundaries of medical knowledge can usefully be interpreted from a neo-Weberian perspective in terms of the competing interests of unorthodox practitioners and the medical establishment in a changing society. As has been seen, the interests of the elite of the medical profession have been particularly influential in this contest over the past two centuries, most recently in strategically limiting the extent of incorporation of unorthodox therapies into mainstream medicine in Britain, through its ongoing dominance of the health care division of labour. This is not to deny, though, the potential value of other perspectives in interpreting the boundary changes involved – as can be illustrated by examples drawn from the Marxist and functionalist approaches to which reference was made at the outset of this chapter.

One key factor which receives particular attention in this area from a Marxist frame of reference is the influence of multinational pharmaceutical corporations in capitalist societies (McKinlay 1985). Such corporations usually possess large-scale resources and spend a substantial proportion of these on promoting drugs by, for instance, distributing free samples, sponsoring medical conferences and advertising in medical journals. This may indeed have helped to induce a medical consciousness more consistent with drug prescription than the use of alternative therapies (Collier 1989) – thus arguably sustaining some of the barriers between orthodox and unorthodox medical knowledge. Similarly, functionalists, in tying the evolving boundary between these forms of knowledge to the needs of the social system, often largely account for its development with reference to the relative efficacy of the therapies which they underpin (see, for example, Wallis and Morley 1976). In this sense, the major success stories of modern medicine, such as the introduction of penicillin and the surgical replacement of faulty heart valves, counterbalanced by the perceived shortcomings of unorthodox medicine in research terms, might be viewed as at least contributing to the explanation of the general tenor of the current relationship between orthodox and unorthodox medicine (Saks 1995).

At the same time, such interpretations need to be treated with caution. Marxist contributors have been prone to overplay the power of the drug companies. In this respect, their forerunners, the newly emergent cluster of small patent medicine businesses, were by no means such a potent force in nineteenth-century British society (Vaughan 1959). The negative influence of the multinational drug companies on unorthodox medicine in the twentieth century, moreover, has for some time been moderated by factors like the increasing diversification of their product range and the financial benefits to be gained from an involvement with alternative therapies given the strength of consumer demand and the limits to the challenge that they pose to biomedical orthodoxy (Saks 1995). The applicability of the functionalist systems approach meanwhile is weakened because it is doubtful whether the medical profession was providing more effective treatment than its competitors when it obtained its monopoly in the mid-nineteenth century, at a stage before aseptic and anaesthetic techniques were systematically introduced and where such questionable methods as bleeding and purging were widely employed (Porter 1987). Equally, the restricted current medical acceptance of unorthodox knowledge is difficult to sustain in light of the counterproductive side-effects of modern medicine and the apparent comparative benefits of unorthodox remedies, particularly for chronic conditions (Pietroni 1991).

The debates about the explanation of the drawing of boundaries between the ideas underlying orthodox and unorthodox health care at any specific point in time will doubtless continue. Further research could certainly be productively conducted into the application of competing perspectives in this field in future. None the less, for the moment the neo-Weberian approach, with its emphasis on interest-based occupational rivalry in a fast changing socio-political context, seems likely to remain of pivotal importance in understanding the fluid boundaries between orthodox and unorthodox medical knowledge in Britain – and particularly the recent qualified shift from 'quackery' to 'complementary' medicine.

References

Alaszewski, A. (1995) 'Restructuring Health and Welfare Professions in the United Kingdom: The Impact of Internal Markets on the Medical, Nursing and Social Work Professions', in T. Johnson, G. Larkin and M. Saks (eds) Health Professions and the State in Europe. London: Routledge.

Bartrip, P. (1990) Mirror of Medicine: A History of the BMJ. Oxford: Clarendon Press.

Berlant, J. L. (1975) Profession and Monopoly: A Study of Medicine in the United States and Great Britain. California: University of California Press.

British Medical Association (1986) Report of the Board of Science and Education on Alternative Therapy. London: BMA.

British Medical Association (1993) Complementary Medicine: New Approaches to Good Practice. Oxford: Oxford University Press.

Brown, P. S. (1985) 'The Vicissitudes of Herbalism in Late Nineteenth and Early Twentieth Century Britain'. Medical History 29: 71–92.

Brown, P. S. (1987) 'Social Context and Medical Theory in the Demarcation of Nineteenth-century Boundaries', in W. F. Bynum and R. Porter (eds) Medical Fringe and Medical Orthodoxy 1750–1850. London: Croom Helm.

Collier, J. (1989) *The Health Conspiracy*. London: Century.

Eagle, R. (1978) *Alternative Medicine*. London: Futura.

Eisenberg, D. M., Kessler, R. C., Foster, C., Norlock, F. E., Calkins, D. R. and Delbanco, T. L. (1993) 'Unconventional Medicine in the United States: Prevalence, Costs, and Patterns of Use'. *New England Journal of Medicine* 328(4): 246–52.

Fulder, S. (1988) *The Handbook of Complementary Medicine*, 2nd edition. Oxford: Oxford University Press.

Fulder, S. and Monro, R. (1981) *The Status of Complementary Medicine in the UK*. London: Threshold Foundation.

Hart, N. (1985) *The Sociology of Health and Medicine*. Ormskirk: Causeway Press.

Inglis, B. (1980) *Natural Medicine*. Glasgow: Fontana.

Jewson, N. (1976) 'The Disappearance of the Sick Man from Medical Cosmology 1770–1870'. *Sociology* 10(2): 225–44.

Larkin, G. (1992) 'Orthodox and Osteopathic Medicine in the Inter-war Years', in M. Saks (ed.) *Alternative Medicine in Britain*. Oxford: Clarendon Press.

Larkin, G. (1995) 'State Control and the Health Professions in the United Kingdom: Historical Perspectives', in T. Johnson, G. Larkin and M. Saks (eds) *Health Professions and the State in Europe*. London: Routledge.

Larkin, G. and Saks, M. (1994) 'Revision or Renewal in the Professional Regulation of Expertise? Relationships Between Orthodox and Unorthodox Medicine'. Paper presented at the International Sociological Association Conference on Regulating Expertise: Professionalism in Comparative Perspective, CERMES, Paris, 14–15 April.

Larner, C. (1992) 'Healing in Pre-industrial Britain', in M. Saks (ed.) *Alternative Medicine in Britain*. Oxford: Clarendon Press.

Lewith, G. and Aldridge, D. (eds) (1991) *Complementary Medicine and the European Community*. Saffron Walden: C.W. Daniel.

Lyng, S. (1990) *Holistic Health and Biomedical Medicine: A Countersystem Analysis*. New York: SUNY Press.

Maple, E. (1992) 'The Great Age of Quackery', in M. Saks (ed.) *Alternative Medicine in Britain*. Oxford: Clarendon Press.

McKee, J. (1988) 'Holistic Health and the Critique of Western Medicine'. *Social Science and Medicine*, 26(8): 775–84.

McKinlay, J. (ed.) (1985) *Issues in the Political Economy of Health Care*. London: Tavistock.

Nicholls, P. A. (1988) *Homoeopathy and the Medical Profession*. London: Croom Helm.

Parssinen, T. (1992) 'Medical Mesmerists in Victorian Britain', in M. Saks (ed.) *Alternative Medicine in Britain*. Oxford: Clarendon Press.

Pietroni, P. (1991) *The Greening of Medicine*. London: Victor Gollancz.

Porter, R. (1987) *Disease, Medicine and Society in England 1550–1860*. London: Macmillan.

Porter, R. (1989) *Health for Sale: Quackery in England 1660–1850*. Manchester: Manchester University Press.

Porter, R. (1994) 'Quacks: An Unconscionable Time Dying', in S. Budd and U. Sharma (eds) *The Healing Bond: The Patient–Practitioner Relationship and Therapeutic Responsibility*. London: Routledge.

Report as to the Practice of Medicine and Surgery by Unqualified Persons in the United Kingdom (1910). London: HMSO.

Saks, M. (1992) 'Introduction', in M. Saks (ed.) *Alternative Medicine in Britain*. Oxford: Clarendon Press.

Saks, M. (1994) 'The Alternatives to Medicine', in J. Gabe, D. Kelleher and G. Williams (eds) *Challenging Medicine*. London: Routledge.

Saks, M. (1995) *Professions and the Public Interest: Medical Power, Altruism and Alternative Medicine*. London: Routledge.

Sharma, U. (1992) *Complementary Medicine Today*: Practitioners and Patients. London: Routledge.

Stacey, M. (1988) *The Sociology of Health and Healing*. London: Unwin Hyman.

Stacey, M. (1992) *Regulating British Medicine: The General Medical Council*. Chichester: John Wiley & Sons.

Vaughan, P. (1959) *Doctors' Commons*. London: Heinemann.

Waddington, I. (1984) *The Medical Profession in the Industrial Revolution*. London: Gill and Macmillan.

Wallis, R. and Morley, P. (1976) 'Introduction', in R. Wallis and P. Morley (eds) *Marginal Medicine*. London: Peter Owen.

Wright, P. (1979) 'A Study in the Legitimisation of Knowledge: The "Success" of Medicine and the "Failure" of Astrology', in R. Wallis (ed.) *On the Margins of Science: The Social Construction of Rejected Knowledge*. Sociological Review Monograph No. 27. Keele: University of Keele.

2 From Charismatic Teaching to Professional Training: The Legitimation of Knowledge and the Creation of Trust in Homoeopathy and Chiropractic

Sarah Cant

Introduction

In 1974, a Druid named Da Monte attracted a dedicated following of non-medically qualified (NMQ) students who wanted to learn and publicize the art of homoeopathy. Despite the absence of formal training structures and qualifications, the students were drawn to the teacher and the knowledge that he could bestow. However, this situation rapidly changed. Within ten years there were several colleges of homoeopathy, curricula, examinations, credentials, a register of qualified practitioners and a code of ethics. These transformations have not been purely organizational; rather, in the space of a decade, the knowledge base of NMQ homoeopathy has been altered and codified. The colleges have engaged in modifications to their training programmes, they have altered the knowledge claims of homoeopathy and have asserted new standards of practice. These changes are not peculiar to homoeopathy and can be witnessed in other complementary therapies. This chapter attempts to account for this shift from the charismatic transmission of knowledge to the development of professional educational practices through an examination of the pressures placed upon alternative therapists to establish external legitimacy and acquire societal trust for their practice.

The sociology of knowledge has established that the content and transmission of knowledge is socially and culturally located (Merton 1957) and that this applies to all forms of learning including lay (Berger and Luckmann 1966), scientific (Woolgar 1981) and medical

(Foucault 1973) knowledge. It is important that the social processes involved in the construction and processes of alternative medical knowledge be subject to the same analysis. Work within the sociology of knowledge has largely been conducted at two broad levels of analysis: first, the social conditions which lead to changes in knowledge; and, second, the activities of those with access to knowledge in terms of their methods of communication and negotiation. This chapter contributes to both these levels through an analysis of NMQ homoeopathy and chiropractic in the UK.

Weber's (1978) concept of charisma will be used as a heuristic device to comprehend ethnographic and historical data on homoeopathy and chiropractic. Weber argued that charisma is an extraordinary quality that is possessed by an individual who, on that account, is then treated as a leader. In this analysis such qualities equip the leader with authority and the power of domination. In this chapter I do not wish to adopt Weber's usage in entirety but instead want to show that the knowledge base of the therapies alone was not enough to explain their revival; rather, the enthusiasm of a select number of teachers created and sustained, for a time, collective excitement about alternative medical ideas. In particular, the early students trusted that their teachers were providing them with a radical new set of ideas. Such a reading can be extracted from Weber who argues that the charismatic leader is obeyed 'by virtue of personal trust in his revelation' (1968: 216).

Weber predicted that charismatic authority would be short-lived and that groups/individuals would tend to claim legitimacy and authority on the basis of rationality and legal/state support. Certainly, throughout the 1980s and 1990s new methods of legitimation for alternative medical knowledge were required. I suggest that charisma could only maintain 'internal' legitimacy and that the personal trust of the students was not sufficient to sustain the alternative medical revival and attract legitimacy from external sources. The sociology of the professions is used to isolate and describe the strategies that have been undertaken to establish a new form of legitimacy and engender this shift from 'personal' to 'societal' trust. The concept of trust is then pivotal to this analysis. Giddens (1994) argues that trust is essential in any situation where knowledge is held by a minority but relied upon by a body of people who are not party to that knowledge. Experts must therefore create and sustain trust between themselves, their knowledge, the lay public and those groups that sanction activity in a society, namely the government and strategic elites (in this case the established medical profession).

The Sociology of the Professions: Trust and Legitimacy

Legitimacy and trust are not automatically created on the basis of the content of a set of knowledge claims, indeed work within the sociology of the professions has established that the ascendance and authority of orthodox medicine was secured by the adoption of a number of professional strategies (also see Saks, this volume). In particular, the medical profession ensured that their knowledge was transmitted to a limited number of practitioners (social closure), who undertook long training to ensure their exclusivity (Parkin 1974) and declared an adherence to the 'scientific' paradigm (Freidson 1970; Larson 1977). Thus, the development of expert and scientific knowledge has been isolated as the prerequisite for the acquisition of high status and a monopoly over medical practice. This monopoly, ensured by support from the state (Johnson 1972), had far-reaching implications for other forms of medical practice. For example, some bodies of knowledge were subject to ridicule and elimination (Wright 1979) and consequently were laid to ground or lost for ever. Another strategy was to co-opt alternative medical knowledges, albeit in altered states, and have orthodox practitioners provide the therapies themselves (Parssinen 1979; Nicholls 1988). Importantly, the incorporation of mesmerism (Parssinen 1979) and homoeopathy (Nicholls 1988), both systems that displayed inconsistency with the contemporary medical paradigm, suggests that orthodox medical practice itself was not internally consistent. In other words, orthodox medical practitioners were prepared to provide alternative forms of medical practice that seemingly contradicted many of the tenets of their own knowledge base. Such a strategy has been explained in terms of self-interest on the part of the medical practitioners who were anxious to retain the support of the public (Saks, this volume), but such a strategy also reveals that the legitimacy of orthodox medical knowledge was not entirely based, as doctors have claimed, on the essential truth, objectivity and coherence of their ideas. Rather, the monopoly wielded by the medical profession came from their ability to diversify their knowledge in practice. Thus, the alternative ideas of medical practice were not simply rejected on the basis of the falsity of their ideas, but sometimes were incorporated into orthodox parameters because they had the potential to compete with orthodox medical practice.

The professionalization of orthodox medicine thus entailed the packaging of their own knowledge base and the manipulation of other medical knowledges. As a result the medical profession secured a position of high authority and legitimacy. It is possible therefore to describe their role as legislative (Bauman 1992) because orthodox practitioners were deemed to have better judgement, superior knowledge and the power to dictate the fate of other knowledges, the latter leading to the suppression of alternative medicine. Larson (1977) suggests that this presentation of expertise, and the financial and status rewards that were acquired by the orthodox practitioners, created an ideology of professionalism, which in turn served to direct the occupational campaigns of other groups.

Within both Weber's analysis of charisma (Parkin 1982) and the sociology of the professions (Esland 1980) there is an assumption that legitimacy also produces authority and power. However, such an equation is not wholly supported as work has pointed to the erosion of the authority of experts, particularly orthodox medical practitioners, through processes of de-professionalization (Haug 1973) and proletarianization (McKinlay and Arches 1985) and such a view has gained some empirical support (Gabe *et al.* 1994). A number of explanations for the demise of absolute authority have been suggested. For example, Bauman (1992) has questioned the durability of authoritative knowledge on the basis of changing relationships with the state and the rise of uncertainty. Giddens (1990; 1991) and Beck (1986) have also highlighted the equation between the development of knowledge and 'risk',[1] and thus an attendant loss of absolute faith in the practice of supposedly rational and scientific knowledge.[2] The evidence of iatrogenic effects associated with the rise of orthodox medical knowledge would support such a view. It is possible then that the emergence of a critique of orthodox medical knowledge (from consumers, the state and the medical profession itself) could have offered alternative medical knowledges an opening in the wider medical market through their own professionalization projects. However, if it is true that knowledge is increasingly regarded as uncertain and risky, it is possible that the rewards of professionalization, as originally secured by the orthodox medical profession, are no longer tenable and that knowledge may not be able to secure a legislative function (Bauman 1992). I want to suggest that alternative medical knowledges, in the light of these wider changes, cannot hope to secure autonomy, authority or secure a monopoly. Nevertheless, the lay public still requires expert knowledge systems and also need to feel secure that their choice of professional is safe and trustworthy. Thus, I argue that the alterations to the mediation and presentation of knowledge have been undertaken to ensure the survival of the therapies and to create a relationship of trust between the practitioners and their consumers and sponsors. The remainder of this chapter documents the shift from 'wisdom' to 'expertise' and the appeal to different forms of legitimacy, but begins with a brief description of homoeopathy and chiropractic.

Homoeopathy and Chiropractic

Homoeopathy was founded by Samuel Hahnemann in the late eighteenth century and is based on principles that are contrary to orthodox medicine. The basic idea is that 'like cures like', that is, the prescription of a remedy to a healthy person would produce the same symptoms as those from which a sick person suffers. The homoeopaths also prescribe highly diluted doses of a remedy, so much so that the original substance is undetectable. The underlying philosophy is that of the vital force, which is conceived as an abstract form of energy which sustains life but may produce illness if weakened. The choice of remedies depends on the specific characteristics of the patient rather than a link to a disease classification (see Sharma, this volume) and consequently prescribing is highly individualized (see Johannessen, this volume).

Homoeopathy is practised in Britain by medically and non-medically qualified (NMQ) or lay homoeopaths. The medically qualified homoeopaths have altered the way that they have practised homoeopathy to sustain the respect of the remainder of the medical profession (Nicholls 1988) and tend to rely upon pathological[3] prescribing for primary care (Cant and Sharma 1996). In this chapter, I focus on one group of NMQ homoeopaths, represented by the Society of Homoeopaths and who currently have 360 licensed members.

Chiropractic is the third largest primary health care profession in the world after medicine and dentistry (Wardwell 1992) and is widely used in the UK (Hansard 1994). As a form of healing it was discovered serendipitously in 1895 by Daniel Palmer who adjusted the vertebrae in his janitor's neck and allegedly cured his long-term deafness. Palmer then developed a theory of disease that suggested misalignment of the vertebrae impinges on the transmission of nerve energy to the vital organs causing organic disease, as well as producing musculo-skeletal problems. Chiropractors locate these misalignments or 'subluxations' and palpate the spine to remove them. Chiropractic was imported to Britain in the 1920s and was practised by a group represented by the British Chiropractic Association. The operation of Common Law in Britain has meant that other practitioners have emerged and there are two other associations currently in existence. The McTimoney Chiropractors, represented by the Institute of Pure Chiropractic and with a membership of 188, is one of these groups and the focus of this chapter.

Methods

The data was collected between 1992 and 1994. Freidson (1986) noted that it is the official representatives of any organization that engage in decision making directed towards occupational development and provide the interface between a group, the lay public and the political economy. Amark (1990) has further noted that the professional association is crucial for the development of knowledge and education. Thus, within homoeopathy and chiropractic, 41 qualitative interviews were conducted with college tutors and representatives from the two professional associations.[4] In addition, six in-depth interviews were undertaken with the first British students in the 1970s' revival of the therapies.

Charismatic Revival

The multifarious and non-sociological use of the term charisma has served to obscure its conceptual and theoretical value (Bensman and Givant 1986; Lindholm 1990). Weber's own work operated at a high level of abstraction (Schnepel 1987) but nevertheless can be applied to the ethnographic data. Following Weber (1978), charisma can be said to exist when a person is treated as a leader and has extraordinary qualities that inspire enthusiasm in his/her followers. Someone with charisma thus engages in relationships that are direct and interpersonal (Gerth and Wright Mills 1986). Using such a definition, we can show the NMQ homoeopaths and McTimoney chiropractors had charismatic revivals in the UK, but that this charisma could only sustain *internal* legitimacy and trust from the followers. This chapter makes no claims about the extent and depth of charismatic authority wielded by each leader.

Within homoeopathy, two Druids, Da Monte and Maughan, independently incorporated homoeopathic healing practices into their Druidic philosophy and attracted a dedicated following from their students:

'Each had a small group of students who were attracted by affinity. And you did not just get homoeopathy but a whole point of view. You just knew that you were getting a huge well of knowledge just by attending his classes. He taught us about the meaning of life and many of us became druids.' (Student)

or

'Well it was different then, not so structured, we learned from a man who was really an esoteric philosopher ... and he used radionics and pendulums ... we had all been treated by him and wanted to learn more.' (Student)

There was no structure to the teaching or a curriculum; rather, these two men would talk about homoeopathy alongside other bodies of knowledge that were far removed from the teachings of medical homoeopathy. There was a great emphasis upon the spirituality of homoeopathy, the vital force and constitutional/individualized prescribing and the students felt they had discovered something that would revolutionize medical practice.

'We wanted to spread this to people because we saw [homoeopathy] having inestimable value and wanted to get people out of the allopathic straitjacket. So the motivating force was love ... we were very euphoric, shall I say about homoeopathy and idealistic. I wanted to shout from the rooftops. Homoeopathy was a vehicle for spiritual change and growth.' (Student)

The homoeopathy that was taught was very different from that practised by medically qualified doctors in Britain, who had taken short, structured and examinable courses by the Faculty. Medical homoeopaths were using the remedies alongside allopathic medicine and were more likely to use pathological prescribing, where a remedy is chosen on the basis of the disease category from which the patient suffers rather than the patient's individual constitution. Lay homoeopathy thus re-emerged as a highly individualistic movement and the teachings further placed great emphasis upon an interactive and non-hierarchical relationship with the patient. There was far more concern about the spread of homoeopathic ideals rather than the accreditation of homoeopathic knowledge and professional training. Thus, there were no stipulations about who could study as it was felt that the best way of expanding the popularity of the approach was to train as many people as possible.

John McTimoney had not had any official tutoring in chiropractic despite its established schools in the US and Bournemouth. After a back complaint of his own in the late 1950s he became fascinated with chiropractic and gradually developed his own techniques. He became a very popular practitioner, with patients apparently queuing down his path in Oxford and who also 'begged' him to teach them his skills. During the 1970s he started to 'pass on' his ideas. As one of his first students reported, 'he was a man of many gifts, a highly individualistic person ... he was unique and he basically taught people in his front room' (Student). Or another describes him as 'an artist, a designer, a healer, he was a wonderful teacher' (Student).

Again, there was no systemic teaching; rather, students would religiously turn up and hear what he had to say. Students found such a practice both exhilarating and daunting.

> 'McTimoney used to go off at tangents and different people were coming in at different times and saying, "train me", and so it went on. There would be people who had done twelve months and then someone else would join and so everyone was at different levels.'
> 'So how long did the training take?'
> 'As long as it took.'

Even if some of the students were discouraged by the haphazard organization they were convinced of the value of chiropractic: 'It was quite different from anything I had ever known before, it was really very valuable.'

In both cases, the teaching was unstructured. The students, drawn by both the teacher and the knowledge that was offered, gained great confidence and dispatched themselves, following a form of apprenticeship, to operate in a 'cottage'[5] industry of medical practice. The teachers emphasized openness and commitment, being less interested in a codified and structured form of knowledge. In turn, these tutors were respected for their wisdom and the students personally trusted their teacher's qualities and abilities to pass on this knowledge. Thus, charisma enabled these therapies to get off the ground (of course other charismatic persons could have done the same) and the teachers stamped their own character upon the knowledge base.

However, in both chiropractic and homoeopathy, the teachers

died and left the students without a knowledge base that could be reproduced. As one homoeopath stated 'we were leaderless, we were desolate'. Moreover, whilst the charisma of the teachers had worked well in the maintenance of 'internal' legitimacy, the death of these 'leaders' coincided with pressures from external bodies for the legitimation of homoeopathic and chiropractic knowledge claims and calls for the groups to establish their trustworthiness. Therefore, to understand the development of alternative medical knowledge systems we must take cognisance of the social pressures upon their claims and organization.

External Pressures for Legitimacy

The last decade has seen mounting external pressures to alter the practice of complementary medicine and an internal recognition by the practitioners of the need to establish boundaries between the qualified practitioner and lay person, to organize internally and to make alterations to the codification and transmission of their knowledge. For example, the government, which took an ambivalent stance towards alternative approaches to health care for many years,[6] has now required that all natural therapies 'get their act together' and has stated that they will contemplate statutory regulation if the therapies prove themselves to be united and well trained. This change of heart by the government is an interesting one and may reflect a concern for the safety of patients or be part of the deregulatory style of government, one that is concerned with cost-effectiveness and competition. Whilst the recent health care reforms have not explicitly referred to complementary medicine, clarification from the Minister for Health in 1991, established that General Practitioners (GPs) could purchase the services of therapists if they wished to orientate their budget in this way (Department of Health 1991). A particular concern also faced the homoeopaths in the guise of the Medicines Act of 1968 which, at the time, was viewed as a threat to the availability of homoeopathic remedies and alerted the practitioners to the need to protect themselves from such legislation by establishing the legitimacy of their approach.

The complementary medical field as a whole was thrown into a panic about the prospect of a common European market and the potential demands from the European Union regarding the harmonization of training standards and knowledge claims across the community. The operation of Napoleonic Law in some European countries restricts much complementary medical practice to ortho-dox doctors (BMA 1993). Whilst it appears that subsidiarity will prevail for the foreseeable future, the various groups within natural medicine have been galvanized to work to protect their position under Common Law.

'We have been able to blossom freely here with Common Law ... but its not like that in other countries, the doctors are very power-ful and they have been pressurising the EC to outlaw non-doctors ... so we need to harmonise our standards.' (Homoeopath)

The influence of the dominant medical profession in the occu-pational development of allied groups has been extensively docu-mented (Donnison 1977; Willis 1992; Witz 1992; Larkin 1983). Until recently the BMA's reaction to complementary medicine has been unfavourable. This was most clearly exhibited in the 1986 BMA report which attempted to discredit the health 'alternatives' as phoney and pseudo-scientific. The latest BMA report (1993) is, however, more favourable and refers to non-orthodox medicine as 'complementary'. The shift in label from alternative to complemen-tary signifies an acceptance that the approaches are no longer anti-thetic but rather 'can work alongside and in conjunction with or-thodox medical treatment' (BMA 1993: 6). Moreover, the BMA has become less interested in whether the therapies work and instead is concerned that they and their patients can be confident of the therapists' professional competence. This rather suggests then that the concern is with the trustworthiness and safety of the practi-tioners rather than the efficacy and content of their knowledge. This change of heart may be in reaction to the failure of the discreditation model and thus the adoption of a model of co-option (Baer 1984; Fairfoot 1987). The BMA also backed the chiropractors' successful claim for statutory regulation in 1994 (HMSO 1994). Whatever the reasoning behind these actions, the BMA has used the report (BMA 1993) as a forum publicly to make demands that the knowledge of complementary therapists be subject to scientific scrutiny, transmitted through proper courses and contain medical science and that orthodox practitioners should retain responsibility for the patient.

Moreover, the consumer through the Association of Community Health Councils (1988) has called for better training and the stand-ardization of curricula and skills. The importance of the user for professionalization has been illustrated (Rothstein 1972; Burrage 1990) and practitioners have recognized the need to orientate themselves to the market and make their knowledge more 'acceptable' to the lay public. Clearly, the small number of practitioners were also concerned to increase the popularity of their approach and could see the advantages of colleges and credentials. Importantly, these external pressures have served as a catalyst for change.

Transforming the Production and Transmission of Knowledge

The death of the leaders of these two groups of alternative practitioners signified a crisis for the legitimacy and future direction of their knowledge and practice. How would their knowledge be sustained and transmitted in the future? In both cases, there were great concerns that the teachings would not survive and it was increasingly recognized that the groups must respond to the demands from the public and the state and protect themselves from European Union rulings and the medical profession. There was a realization that the groups needed to distinguish themselves from the lay public and the criticism that they were untrained and unsafe. To be able to make such a case for their legitimacy required that changes be made to their knowledge. Specifically, it was important that they could be clear about what constituted and demarcated homoeopathic and chiropractic knowledge. Thus, both groups independently came to the decision that their teachings had to acquire an 'authenticity'. The changes made to the knowledge can be divided into four areas: codification and accreditation, tempering of knowledge claims, alignment to science, and the creation of boundaries around who can exercise the knowledge. The alterations resemble the professionalization process of orthodox medicine undertaken in the late nineteenth century.

Codification and Accreditation

The most immediate concern for the students of homoeopathy and chiropractic was to ensure that the knowledge they had acquired would not be lost. In both cases a college and professional association was established with the aim to establish a curriculum and an educational institution that would be attractive to a wider body of students. McTimoney chiropractic still has only one college, whilst NMQ homoeopathy has expanded greatly and currently has 21 colleges. Whilst there are some differences amongst the colleges, the Society of Homoeopaths, established in 1981, has stipulated the prerequisites of a core curriculum, will only recommend to students courses that meet these criteria and has ensured the systematization of the teaching. As one homoeopath stated, 'We have moved on tremendously from the early days, we compare very favourably to a university undergraduate degree' (Society member and College Principal).

Naturally the knowledge base of these therapies did not become conterminous with the core curriculum, but there have been serious attempts to codify the knowledge so that it can be passed on in a structured way. The retention of the principle that patients be seen as individuals now sits alongside the systematic teaching of the repertory and the organon, in the case of homoeopathy, and the mechanics of the body in the case of chiropractic. Moreover, students who successfully complete the courses receive qualifications and can join a register of qualified practitioners that is guaranteed by the professional association. Such accreditation is fundamental to the acquisition of a trust relationship because the possession of credentials provides a cultural currency that speaks of safety and trustworthiness. The chiropractors successfully gained statutory regulation in 1994, whereby only properly qualified practitioners are allowed to call themselves chiropractors, and this provides their training with legal status. Such recognition was only possible, however, once their training had been shown to be detailed and have the unanimous support of all chiropractic groups (Hansard 1994).

Tempering of Knowledge Claims

The early teachings within both groups alerted students to the wide-ranging potential of their discipline. There was an espousal of the holism of their 'art' and a suggestion that other forms of medical care, particularly orthodox medicine, would gradually become redundant. Within chiropractic it was believed that the manipulation of the spine had the potential to cure the whole range of mechanical and organic problems, and the Druidic homoeopaths stressed the danger of orthodox medicine, the spirituality of the vital force and the ability of homoeopathy to deal with all medical problems. However, throughout the 1980s we have witnessed the gradual curtailment of these ideals.

Within homoeopathy, the Druidic and esoteric components of the teaching have been largely jettisoned in the public portrayal of the therapy. Practitioners may use crystals or employ the use of the pendulum to aid the choice of remedy and engage in research about links with other bodies of knowledge (see Sharma, this volume), but the discussion of these areas is confined to the in-house journals and is not mentioned in public literature. The directors of the Society of Homoeopaths are also anxious to phrase their knowledge claims in an acceptable way and try to avoid talking of the vital force. 'We don't talk about the vital force, especially when talking to doctors, we might mention magnetic fields and that sort of stuff' (Officer of Society).

Chiropractic had attracted a great deal of scepticism because of the original broad scope of practice. However, during the last ten years, especially throughout the campaign for statutory regulation, we have seen the group emphasize and develop the musculo-skeletal side of their therapy.

Moreover, both groups publicly state that their practice should not be regarded as alternative but, rather, complementary to orthodox medicine. This change in emphasis can be seen as a conscious alteration to the type of knowledge that is deemed acceptable and the type of public messages that the practitioners are prepared to make. For example, within homoeopathy, it has been decided that practitioners must no longer advise their patients to reject vaccinations. Similarly, a leaflet from the professional association that criticizes vaccinations has been withdrawn, 'We had to ask whether it was in our professional interests to cover this area ... we were beginning to see it was not our function to give out this advice' (Society member).

Alignment to the Scientific Paradigm

The professional project and the attendant acquisition of legitimacy has been linked to the development of scientific knowledge (Freidson 1970; Larson 1977). In homoeopathy and chiropractic the legacy of broad claims for their therapies and the inconsistency of their knowledge base in comparison to orthodox medical science has had the potential to stand as an obstacle to recognition. Thus, both groups have made consistent efforts to attach their knowledge *publicly* to the scientific paradigm (such an enterprise is not necessarily followed within the therapies). These efforts have operated at three levels. First, all the colleges have incorporated medical science into their curriculums and conceive of biology, pathology and physiology as constituent parts of their knowledge system.

'We spend a whole year on anatomy and physiology and then three years looking at pathology, the best colleges would maintain they offer an equivalent to a medical degree.' (College Principal in Homoeopathy)

Second, the groups have attempted to use scientific theories to try and explain why their therapy works. This has been less successful for the homoeopaths, who despite attempts to use biophysics as an explanatory framework, have yet to produce an agreed theory of the law of similars.[7] Chiropractic has, however, had more success, in particular through the application of orthopaedic principles to explain the operation of chiropractic.

Third, the chiropractors and medically qualified homoeopaths have used scientific procedures, particularly randomized control trials to establish that their therapy works in practice (Reilly *et al.* 1986; Meade *et al.* 1990). The NMQ homoeopaths have yet to employ such a procedure, partly because of the expense of launching a trial, but there is an increasing commitment to such methods from the Society, even if such a sentiment is not held by all members.

Boundary Construction

Originally, as we have seen, both forms of medical practice were very open. As one homoeopath stated:

'We had discovered and had been part of a system that was truly wonderful, really and truly wonderful and the fire was there, we wanted to get it to others ... so that was the motivating force, get it to everybody.'

However, it was recognized by the politically active members of both groups that external legitimacy could only be achieved if a case could be made for the expertise and specialism of the practitioners. In other words they recognized the need to close off their knowledge. Such closure is made possible by higher entry requirements and longer training programmes (Weber 1968). In homoeopathy, the courses now run over four years part-time with a fifth year of supervised clinical practice, and the McTimoney chiropractic course lasts three years. Recommendations have also been made about entry requirements, although these do not necessarily operate in practice. For example, the Society of Homoeopaths suggests students should have two A-levels but they will accept entrants with relevant life experience on to their courses.

The establishment of registers of qualified practitioners has also served to demarcate the 'authentic' practitioner from one that simply calls him/herself a chiropractor or homoeopath as permitted by the conditions of Common Law. Once on the register, the practitioners have proved that they have passed their examinations and supervised practice and that they have agreed to conform to a strict code of ethics. Any violation of the code of ethics can involve the practitioners being struck off the register. This attachment to credentials and registration appears to have been introduced for external purposes, for, interestingly, within the homoeopathic organization there are few attempts to exert authority or establish hierarchies and much emphasis is placed upon co-operation and equality.

Dilemmas

The picture painted of the groups' attempts to change the content and transmission of their knowledge and alter their practice appears very straightforward and unproblematic. However, in reality the transition has not been altogether smooth. Concerns revolve around the issues of exclusivity, the loss of the intrinsic qualities of the therapy, the fear of subordination to orthodox authority and practice, and the inappropriateness of the scientific paradigm. First, then, some of the original students balk at the developments, in particular the idea of restricting the practice of the therapy to a few highly educated individuals. This complaint is most apparent in homoeopathy with some practitioners suggesting that their practice has become everything that they once deplored. For example, the development of 'expertise' is thought by some as contrary to the original principles of a non-hierarchical and participative therapy, with both practitioner and patient involved in the healing process. Second, and not unrelated to the first point, there are concerns that the real essence and the individuality of these alternative approaches to medicine have been lost. As one homoeopath stated:

'They have dumped the training we got from Thomas Maughan, they have shifted and tried to seek respectability ... I want nothing to do with that because it destroys our ideals.' (Society member)

Third, the groups are concerned that by accepting a complementary role for their practice they may have served to subordinate their knowledge to that of orthodox medicine. Certainly, whilst the chiropractors have received statutory regulation (HMSO 1994), this has not secured them any autonomy, or rights to educational grants, or payment through the NHS. On the contrary, their practice is confined to the private sector, their scope of intervention has been defined publicly as musculo-skeletal complaints and they have agreed that orthodox doctors retain responsibility for the patient[8] (Cant and Sharma 1994). In other words the strategies of professionalization have not rewarded the groups with autonomy or a monopoly of practice. Similarly, factions within homoeopathy feel that they may have secured their survival, but they have cast themselves as a profession supplementary to orthodox medicine, and as a therapy that has lost its potential. As one homoeopath stated:

'Homoeopathy is a vehicle for spiritual change and growth. [The students] now come out seeing themselves as remedy givers or doctors, they have dumped the idea of homoeopathy as an evolutionary tool of development.' (Society member)

and another lamented that

'homoeopathy (will) have ceased to teach our insights to the medically destructive mind of the world.' (Society member)

Similarly, some homoeopaths feel that statutory regulation will curtail diversity, encourage the re-emergence of a medical monopoly and constitute 'sleeping with the enemy' (Kirk 1994: 6).

Finally, the alignment to the scientific paradigm has been seen as problematic. For example, some chiropractors feel that the use of orthopaedic science has served to explain away many valuable aspects of their therapy, especially the treatment of organic illness. The homoeopaths still continue to experiment with other bodies of knowledge and in so doing extend their own knowledge (see Sharma, this volume) but recognize that scientific-based knowledge is important for legitimacy and recognition.

Therefore, whilst the professional organizations have engaged in a professional project on behalf of their members, there are many internal contradictions which have yet to be resolved. Consequently, the concern to assert the legitimacy of chiropractic and homoeopathy in the public arena has often been at odds with the wishes of the grassroots practitioners.

Conclusions

During the last twenty years the homoeopaths and chiropractors have engaged in alterations to their knowledge production and transmission. The codification of knowledge, the abandonment of informal modes of knowing and learning, the limitation of access and the alignment to the scientific paradigm have provided the groups with an external legitimacy based on their professionalism. Yet, this shift from charismatic leadership and teaching, which inspired commitment and following, to professional training has been in direct contradiction to many of the original principles of these therapies. Moreover, it was these early principles that made homoeopathy and chiropractic attractive to patients and students in the 1970s. Evidence about the use of alternative medicine suggests that some of the attraction for the therapies comes from a desire for increased participation in the healing process and greater attention to the social and spiritual dimensions of health care (Bakx 1991; Cant and Calnan 1991; Sharma 1992), as well as more pragmatic demands for more time from the practitioner and less interventionist methods (Thomas et al. 1991). It is possible then that such transformations may serve to reduce the appeal of these healing approaches.

Nevertheless, the alterations made to the knowledge bases have had some positive effects. We have seen that the BMA became more favourably disposed to these alternatives once they were able to exhibit professional competence. Similarly, the government was prepared to offer statutory regulation to both osteopathy (HMSO 1993) and chiropractic (HMSO 1994) once they could prove the strength of their teaching and practice. It appears that the legitimacy of these groups has been won less on the basis of the content of their knowledge and more on the presentation and organization of their educational practices and knowledge claims. Indeed, when the BMA was interested only in the actual content of the knowledge claims of alternative medicine (BMA 1986), the approaches were condemned as quackery. The legitimacy of alternative medical knowledge thus seems to have been achieved through the establishment of a relationship of trust between the practitioners and their consumers and sponsors, based on the transmission and presentation of their knowledge.

However, the professional project of homoeopathy and chiropractic has not delivered any traditional rewards. The groups have not been able to secure a monopoly of practice. Whilst it is now illegal for non-approved persons to call themselves a chiropractor, there is nothing in law stopping someone providing the same techniques but under another title, for example, bonesetter. It is unlikely that the groups will attain further autonomy, indeed it is possible that they may in fact now have fewer freedoms than they wielded in the 1970s. For example, under the conditions of Common Law, anyone can practise a form of medical practice as long as they do not call themselves a doctor. This freedom allowed the legal revival of these therapies, and practitioners could work fairly autonomously without recourse to medical opinion. Now the groups have accepted a position of complementarity to orthodox medicine and largely accept medical authority. Indeed the BMA report (1993) states that medical practitioners should be informed of all other forms of care and should retain ultimate responsibility for the patient. It is also unclear whether the groups have acquired higher status. Certainly, the recognition from the government provided by the Chiropractors Act (HMSO 1994) is an advance and is desired by the homoeopaths, however, there a few financial rewards to be earned as the practitioners have not secured a position within the NHS. It could be argued that such a right would not be beneficial and that there is more money to be made in the private sector. Such an argument would hold for the chiropractors – the practitioners I spoke to were very well paid. However, it is not possible to extrapolate such a finding to other groups. Many of the homoeopaths were poorly paid,[9] had other jobs to supplement their salary and were unable to structure their financial situation as they could not predict or stabilize their earnings.

The description and analysis of these changes within alternative medical knowledge points to the importance of the social context for the shape and fate of knowledge systems. The therapists really had very little choice but to attend to the organization and transmission of their knowledge if they wanted the support of the state, the medical profession and their consumers. The process of change was thus dynamic, involving the interaction between the interests of the practitioners and those that surrounded them. This chapter has also pointed to the actual strategies and forms of negotiation that were applied. In the past such strategies secured positions of high status and financial reward. However, societal belief in the absolute authority of expert knowledge has been eroded (Beck 1986; Giddens 1994). Instead, I suggest, groups can only work to retain the trust of their users, and it is here that the strategies of professionalization still appear to be salient. As alternative medical knowledge extended its popularity and attracted interest from outside bodies, the internal legitimacy and personal trust of the charismatic leaders could not sustain the credibility of these knowledge systems; instead, strategies of professionalization, including the alignment to science, were undertaken in a bid to secure wider societal legitimacy and trust. Consequently, debates about the fragmentation of knowledge and the collapse of the metanarrative (Lyotard 1986; Introduction, this volume) do not hold true in the *public* representations of these therapies. Internally, groups may be committed to pluralism and eclecticism, but the award of legitimacy still hinges on a pretence, at least, to the scientific paradigm.

Acknowledgements

I would like to thank Tim Fox for his support.

Notes

1. It is suggested in late modernity that unintended consequences result from the development of knowledge. Knowledge does not simply deliver advantage and progress but also the potential for risk and danger.
2. The magnification of risks associated with the rise of orthodox medicine has been documented (Illich 1975; Gabe *et al.* 1994).
3. Prescribing on the basis of a disease classification.
4. The project was generously funded by the Economic and Social Science Research Council. The project was undertaken with Ursula Sharma and I am grateful for her extensive support and encouragement.
5. The practitioners tended to work alone and survive by attracting their own local and often dedicated patients.
6. Evidenced by the operation of Common Law in the UK. The government has not always acted in the favour of the medical profession, spiritual healers were allowed to work in the NHS in the 1970s and 1991 saw the clarification that GPs could purchase the services of complementary therapists.
7. Sharma in this volume shows that internally there are many more various efforts to make sense of homoeopathy.
8. This latter principle is also established in the BMA report for all complementary practitioners.
9. A recent survey by the Society confirmed that the majority of homoeopaths earn less than £5000 per annum (Newsletter 1995).

References

Amark, K. (1990) 'Open Cartels and Social Closures: Professional Strategies in Sweden, 1860–1950', in M. Burrage and R. Torstendahl, *Professions in Theory and History*. London: Sage.

Association of Community Health Councils (1988) *The State of Non-Conventional Medicine – The Consumer View*. London: ACHC.

Baer, H. (1984) 'The Drive for Professionalization in British Osteopathy'. *Social Science and Medicine* 19(7): 717–25.

Bakx, K. (1991) 'The Eclipse of Folk Medicine in Western Society'. *Sociology of Health and Illness*, 13(1): 20–38.

Bauman, Z. (1992) *Intimations of Modernity*. London: Routledge.

Beck, U. (1986) *Risk Society. Towards a New Modernity*. London: Sage.

Bensman, J. and Givant, M. (1986) 'Charisma and Modernity: The Use and Abuse of a Concept', in R. Glassman and W. Swatos (eds) *Charisma, History and Social Structure*. London: Greenwood Press.

Berger, P. and Luckmann, T. (1966) *The Social Construction of Reality*. London: Penguin.

BMA (1986) *Alternative Therapy. Report of the Board of Science and Education*. London: BMA.

BMA (1993) *Complementary Medicine. New Approaches to Good Practice*. Oxford: Oxford University Press.

Burrage, M. (1990) 'Introduction: The Professions in Sociology and History', in M. Burrage and R. Torstandahl, *Professions in Theory and History*. London: Sage.

Cant, S. and Calnan, M. (1991) 'On the Margins of the Medical Marketplace? An Exploratory Study of Alternative Practitioners Perceptions'. *Sociology of Health and Illness* 13(1): 39–57.

Cant, S. and Sharma, U. (1994) *Professionalization in Complementary Medicine*. Final Report to the Economic and Social Research Council.

Cant, S. and Sharma, U. (1996) 'Demarcation and Transformation Within Homoeopathic Knowledge. A Strategy of Professionalization'. *Social Science and Medicine* 42(4): 579–88.

Department of Health (1991) 'Stephen Dorrell Clarifies the Position on Alternative and Complementary Medicine'. Press Release, 3 December 1991.

Donnison, J. (1977) *Midwives and Medical Men*. London: Heinemann.

Esland, G. (1980) 'Professions and Professionalism', in G. Esland and G. Salaman, *The Politics of Work and Occupations*. Milton Keynes: Open University Press.

Fairfoot, P. (1987) 'Alternative Therapies. The BMA Knows Best', *Journal of Social Policy* 16: 383–90.

Freidson, E. (1970) *Profession of Medicine*. Chicago: University of Chicago Press.

Freidson, E. (1986) *Professional Powers: A Study of the Institutionalization of Formal Knowledge*. Chicago and London: University of Chicago Press.

Foucault, M. (1973) The Birth of The Clinic. London: Routledge.
Gabe, J., Kelleher, D. and Williams, G. (1994) Challenging Medicine. London: Routledge.
Gerth, H. and Wright Mills, C. (1986) 'Bureaucracy and Charisma', in R. Glassman and W. Swatos (eds) Charisma, History and Social Structure. London: Greenwood Press.
Giddens, A. (1990) The Consequences of Modernity. Oxford: Polity Press.
Giddens, A. (1991) Modernity and Self Identity. Oxford: Polity Press.
Giddens, A. (1994) 'Living in a Post-Traditional Society', in U. Beck, A. Giddens and S. Lash (1994) Reflexive Modernization. Oxford: Polity Press.
Haug, M. (1973) 'De-professionalization: An Alternative Hypothesis for the Future'. Sociological Review Monograph 20: 195–211.
Hansard (1994) 'Chiropractors Bill', 18 February 1994.
HMSO (1993) The Osteopaths Act. London: HMSO.
HMSO (1994) The Chiropractic Act. London: HMSO.
Illich, I. (1975) Medical Nemesis. London: Calder and Boyars.
Johnson, T. (1972) Professions and Power. London: Macmillan.
Kirk, A (1994) 'The Alternative to Being Alternative. Some Contributions to the State Registration Debate'. The Society of Homoeopaths Newsletter, September 1994.
Larkin, G. (1983) Occupational Monopoly and Modern Medicine. London: Tavistock.
Larson, M. S. (1977) The Rise of Professionalism: A Sociological Analysis. Los Angeles: California University Press.
Lindholm, C. (1990) Charisma. Oxford: Blackwell.
Lyotard, J. (1980) The Postmodern Condition: A Report on Knowledge. Manchester: Manchester University Press.
McKinlay, J. and Arches, J. (1985) 'Towards the Proletarianization of Physicians'. International Journal of Health Services 15: 161–95.
Meade, T. W., Dyer, S., Browne, W., Townsend, J. and Frank, A. O. (1990) 'Low Back Pain of Mechanical Origin: Randomised Comparison of Chiropractic and Hospital Out-Patient Treatment'. BMJ 300(2): 1431–7, June 1990.
Merton, R. K. (1957) Social Theory and Social Structure. New York: Free Press.
Nicholls, P. (1988) Homoeopathy and the Medical Profession. London: Croom Helm.
Parkin, F. (1974) The Social Analysis of Class Structure. London: Tavistock.
Parkin, F. (1982) Max Weber. London: Tavistock.
Parssinen, T. (1979) 'Professional Deviants and the History of Medicine: Medical Mesmerists in Victorian Britain', in R. Wallis (ed.) Sociological Review Monograph 27: 103–21.
Reilly, D. T., Taylor, M. A.., McSharry, C. and Aitkinson, T. (1986) 'Is Homoeopathy a Placebo Response? Controlled Trial of Homoeopathic Potency, with Pollen in Hayfever as a Model'. Lancet 287: 337–9.
Rothstein, W. (1972) American Physicians in the Nineteenth Century.

Baltimore: Johns Hopkins University Press.

Schnepel, B. (1987) 'Max Weber's Theory of Charisma and its applicability to Anthropological Research'. *Journal of the Anthropological Society in Oxford* 18(1): 26–48.

Sharma, U. (1992) *Complementary Medicine Today. Practitioners and Patients*. London: Routledge.

Thomas, K., Carr, J., Westlake, L. and Williams, B. (1991) 'Use of Non-orthodox and Conventional Health Care in Great Britain'. *BMJ* 302: 207–10.

Wardwell, W. (1992) *History and Evolution of a New Profession*. St Louis, MO: Mosby Year Book.

Weber, M. (1968) *Economy and Society*, G. Roth and C. Wittich (eds). New York: Bedminster Press.

Weber, M. (1978) *Economy and Society*. London: University of California Press.

Willis, E. (1992) *Medical Dominance*. Sydney: Allen and Unwin.

Witz, A. (1992) *Professions and Patriarchy*. London: Routledge.

Wright, P. W. G. (1979) 'A Study in the Legitimation of Knowledge: The "Success" of Medicine and the "Failure" of Astrology', in R. Wallis (ed.) *Sociological Review Monograph* 27: 103–21.

Woolgar, S. (1981) 'Interests and Explanation in the Social Study of Science'. *Social Studies of Science* 11(3): 365–94.

3 The Comfrey Controversy

Midge Whitelegg

Comfrey is a herb much used and loved by herbalists. Its use has been severely curtailed in recent years as far afield as Canada and Australia as well as in Europe, and European Union (EU) legislation may threaten it further. It is important to look at the circumstances giving rise to the limitations, for the conflict therein embodies a much wider debate that is fundamental to the relationship between orthodox and complementary medicine as a whole. In this chapter, I shall discuss the controversy about the herb comfrey in terms of two main themes. First, my argument is based upon the Kuhnian notion of paradigms and suggests a perspective of complementary medicine representing a paradigmatic alternative to orthodox medicine – namely that complementary medicine offers a different tradition and culture in which healing can take place, and, if pressed, might articulate a different notion of science involving, among other things, admission of uncertainty and collaborative generation of knowledge. Kuhn's (1970) premise of incommensurability of paradigms – the one cannot be measured by the yardstick of the other – is crucial. Second, the concept of science as certainty is questioned and the coherence of the scientific argument within its own terms addressed.

Kuhn described a paradigm as a set of assumptions defined by a particular methodology, shared by a group working in a particular area. A paradigm becomes dominant because it enables a set of problems to be solved. Once the status of dominant paradigm has been achieved, its basic tenets are taken for granted, allowing scientists to avoid starting from first principles in their researches. 'Normal science' solves problems within the paradigm: 'its object is to solve a puzzle for whose very existence the validity of the paradigm must be assumed' (Kuhn 1970: 80). It does not aim to produce novelties that question the paradigm itself: 'no part of the aim of normal science is to call forth new sorts of phenomena; indeed those that will not fit the box are often not seen at all' (Kuhn 1970: 24).

If a paradigm is to change, challenged by a new candidate for dominant paradigm, it can only happen through revolution and the consequences are profound. Seeing nature in a completely different way, there is a shift in the entire conception of science, the problems it addresses and the application of associated methodologies. I suggest that beliefs within herbal medicine can be constituted in a different paradigm from orthodox medicine and the comfrey controversy can be articulated in this context, rather than simply representing a substantial disagreement within the dominant paradigm, in that complementary medicine offers a different notion of science involving, among other things, a move from strict reductionism, intrusion of an amount of subjectivity, contextualization of knowledge and admission of uncertainty. Conflicting paradigms, Kuhn maintains, are incompatible in that the conflict cannot be resolved by recourse to the tenets of the paradigms because they will inevitably disagree about what is a problem and its solution; they are necessarily incommensurable.

Kuhn has been criticized on a number of counts. Mulkay (1972), while not denying that revolutions occur, suggested intellectual migration as a more likely route to innovation. This possibility is considered elsewhere (Whitelegg 1995). Barnes (1982) expresses frustration at the lack of explanation for scientists' behaviour in Kuhn's work. Developments in the sociology of scientific knowledge have taken Kuhn's ideas further and have questioned the objective nature of science. Saks supports the interests approach in this volume.

Herbalists' training includes orthodox sciences, diagnosis and examination. They nevertheless undertake a treatment strategy that embraces the individual in as entire a context as possible and actively seek to involve the patient in the healing process. The herbalist must know the active constituents of the plants they use, and how the whole plant behaves – often differently – in the body. Investigations are valued and usually affirm traditional usage. Clinical trials too are consulted, yet some can prove of limited use when the testing of one herb, for example, over a large number of people may not be a sufficiently precise indication of its use in context – is feverfew, for example, better in 'hot' migraines or 'cold' ones (Mills 1991), and is it better not to use it in migraines with an amount of debility (McIntyre 1995), and how does it behave differently when mixed with a choice from the other 200 or so popular herbs for any one prescription containing on average four or five; moreover, in this context, what 'type' of person will it best suit, and how might, for example, patient attitude influence its effect? Further herbal knowledge is gained through study of traditional usage in native European and wider cultures, amplified by the experience of practising herbalists accessed both through literature and in the form of a minimum of 500 hours' clinical training/apprenticeship with mentor herbalists undertaken towards the end of formal training. They are encouraged to develop, through thorough knowledge of herbs and keen observation of people, an amount of intuitive practice.

In this chapter I suggest that the arguments against comfrey are spoken from an orthodox paradigm, but that the paradigm is inappropriate and the arguments flawed within it. I leave it to the reader to impute the motives. In discussing the comfrey issue I look at the use of the plant and summarise the case against it. I then look more closely at some of the major papers making the arguments against comfrey and the strategies employed by orthodoxy to consolidate the case against it and in support of banning its use. The rigour of orthodox science is questioned and the appropriateness of its use for measuring an alternative paradigm is addressed.

The Herb

Comfrey or Symphytum belongs to the family Boraginaceae. There are a number of species within the Symphytum genus, the two implicated here are Symphytum officinale and upplandicum. S. upplandicum is a hybrid of officinale and asperum and is called Russian comfrey. Comfrey is known by other names, such as knitbone, boneset, bruisewort, or consormol. Symphytum derives from the Greek *symphyo*, indicating its gluing properties. Its Latin name was *consolida*, from the verb *consolidare* – to glue together or close – hence too the old English *consound* and the French *consoude*. Comfrey is from the Latin *confirmare*, meaning to heal or unite. Knitbone and the German *Beinwell* both refer to the plant's abilities to heal fractures. Parts used are fresh or dried leaves or roots.

Its constituents include mucilage, allantoin, tannins, resin, essential oil, pyrrolizidine alkaloids, gum, carotene, glycosides, sugars, beta-sitosterol and steroidal saponins, triterpenoids, vitamin B12, protein and zinc. Main culinary uses are the fresh leaves and shoots as vegetable or salad while for medicinal purposes, according to the *British Herbal Pharmacopoeia*:

Actions: vulnerary. demulcent. anti-haemorrhagic. anti-rheumatic. anti-inflammatory.

Indications: gastritis and duodenal ulcer. Rheumatic pain. Arthritis. Topically as poultice or fomentation in bruises, sprains, athlete's foot, crural ulcer and mastitis.

Specific indication: gastric ulcer. Topically varicose ulcer.

(British Herbal Medicine Association 1985: 202–3)

Other recent herbals describe its properties. McIntyre, former president of the National Institute of Medical Herbalists (NIMH) says:

Comfrey is one of the most famed healing plants. Its remarkable power to heal tissue and bone is due to allantoin, a cell proliferant that promotes the growth of connective tissue, bone and cartilage, and is easily absorbed through the skin ... useful as a poultice for varicose ulcers and a compress for varicose veins ... alleviates and heals minor burns ... traditional remedy for gastric ulcers ... used to treat colitis ... useful for bronchitis and other respiratory disorders. (McIntyre 1988: 33)

Perhaps Culpepper's description of the vulnerary properties of the root is the most lurid: '... if they be boiled with dissevered pieces of flesh in a pot, it will join them together again' (Culpepper 1979: 43).

It is important to note that an essential part of the herbalists' creed is to use whole plants in the form of teas or tinctures, for example. Individual chemicals are never extracted for use in isolation. Herbalists believe that the chemicals in a particular plant act synergistically, making the action of the plant more than the sum of its individual parts. The alkaloid ephedrine from the plant Ephedra, for example, proved, for the pharmaceutical companies, unusable in isolation, because of its hypertensive effects. Further investigation of the whole plant revealed another alkaloid, pseudo-ephedrine, with the capacity to reduce blood pressure, rendering the plant safer in its entirety. In addition the NIMH has a specific policy, passionately defended, of not experimenting on animals in any circumstances.

The Controversy

The controversy arises in relation to the pyrrolizidine alkaloids (PAs) found in the comfrey root and to a lesser extent in the leaves. Similar alkaloids are found in other species of plant, and have been found toxic to both humans and animals. As reports in the scientific literature and the media demonstrating the harmful effects built up, demands that comfrey be banned increased. It is currently banned in Canada, Germany and Australia. In the UK the internal use of the root, and any tablets containing leaf or root, are considered harmful. Use of the leaf is still permitted, but EU legislation is pending.

Pyrrolizidine alkaloids have been implicated in numerous cases of poisoning in humans and animals.

Poisoning in Animals

Both acute and chronic toxicity has been observed in animals in the field and the laboratory. Bone (n.d.) cites Maclean who reports liver, lung, nerve, gastric and kidney damage in field animals. According to Culvenor *et al.* (1980) citing Schoental, in laboratory rats tumours have been found in the liver, lung, kidney, gastro-intestinal tract, brain, spinal cord and pancreas as a result of pyrrolizidine poisoning. Tests have also been conducted on mice, hamsters, guinea pigs, rabbits, monkeys, sheep, chickens and quail – the effect varying with each species, Pembery (1982) reports, citing Mattocks.

Poisoning in Humans

Poisoning in humans manifests as veno-occlusive disease of the liver detected by microscopic examination. PA poisoning occurs either from food contamination or from ingestion of herbs as medicine in the form of teas or, more recently, capsules.

The disease is endemic in Jamaica where the drinking of large quantities of 'bush teas' containing Senecio or Crotelaria species is usual. Culvenor *et al.* (1980) give examples of PA poisoning. They cite Datta *et al.* reporting three cases of hepatic veno-occlusive disease in the 1970s from consumption of Heliotropium eichwaldi as a medicinal herb in India. Culvenor *et al.* (1980) also mention Dubrovinskii's reports on epidemics in the USSR from 1935 to the mid-1950s through contamination of bread made from wheat, barley or millet containing Heliotropium lasiocarpum. Four Chinese women developed liver disease after taking a herbal tea for psoriasis (Kumana *et al.* 1985). In an epidemic in Afghanistan 1630 people in one area were affected by contaminated flour, again containing Heliotropium (Mohabbat *et al.* 1976). The list is long.

As a result of these and other cases, repeated calls that comfrey be banned have appeared in the literature. Even the Henry Doubleday Institute issued a statement in 1978, reported in the *British Medical Journal* (BMJ) 1979, which concluded that until further research clarifies the long-term health hazard of comfrey ingestion, 'no human being or animal should eat, drink, or take Comfrey in any form' (*BMJ* 1979: 598). Given the above data, it is surprising rather that comfrey has only recently been restricted. But on closer inspection the case is not so overwhelmingly negative.

A Closer Look

Toxicity in Animals

Take the first premise that comfrey is toxic to animals. Cases of poisoning in field animals have been caused by PAs from species other than comfrey. Hills, in his introduction to Pembery's report for the Doubleday Institute 1982, revoking their previous warning, says:

> The Commonwealth Bureau of Animal Health very kindly carried out a computer search through their records of 137,000 cases of stock poisoning by plants since 1972 and found only one concerning comfrey-nitrate poisoning in pigs from excessive use of fertiliser in Germany. (Pembery 1982: 6)

Reports in the later scientific literature concern themselves more with laboratory animals where testing can be controlled. One of the main champions of the PA poisoning hypothesis is Culvenor in Australia. He has published a number of papers on the effects of PA poisoning on rats. In the paper 'The structure and toxicology of the alkaloids of Russian Comfrey, a medicinal herb and item of human diet' (Culvenor et al. 1980), he reported on an experiment in which alkaloids of comfrey were administered intraperitoneally to two-week-old rats either as a single dose or as multiple doses beginning at two weeks old over intervals of nine weeks. Evidence of hepatotoxicity was found. Bone (n.d.) and Pembery (1982) both make closer investigations. They both suggest that two-week-old rats are more vulnerable to the effects of PAs and, according to Jago (1971), are particularly susceptible to the induction of megalocytosis. Pembery looks carefully at the numerical data and extrapolates quantities for humans by analogy. He continues:

it can be seen that the dose required to produce the least effect in the rats, i.e. reduced liver function, detectable by a change in the proportion of the plasma proteins, is equivalent to the alkaloid from 5607 leaves if administered to a 'man sized' [sic] rat. That is, if we assume that the effect of the alkaloid in man is going to be the same as in a young rat, apparently the most susceptible of any so far tested. If an average comfrey leaf is taken as 100g (and older leaves are much more than this), this dose level represents about eight times the body weight of the 'man sized' rat. Deaths occurred at levels equivalent to the alkaloid from 19,880 leaves or equivalent to 28 times the body weight of the 'man sized' rat. (Pembury 1982: 13)

Most importantly, however, both papers argue that to give alkaloids in isolation and injected peritoneally into animals cannot reflect the effects in humans of the entire plant taken orally. A rejoinder from the NIMH replying to a number of attacks speaks of:

two insupportable assumptions. First, that the naturally occurring complex in the plant ... can be regarded as a mere physical dilution of alkaloids and secondly, that the human metabolism is identical with that of the rat which is susceptible to these alkaloids, and not with the sheep which is resistant to them. (NIMH 1982: 1)

The NIMH makes a further point:

Tea, almonds, apples, pears, mustard, radishes and hops, to list only a few items, all contain substances which, if extracted, can be shown to be poisonous when tested under conditions similar to those used in the comfrey experiments. Must we then ignore our experience of the usefulness and wholesomeness of these foods because controlled trials and scientific evidence have not been published to establish their safety. (NIMH 1982: 1)

This example serves to highlight an aspect of the fundamental clash of paradigms between orthodox and alternative medicine: orthodoxy, on the one hand, demanding scientific proof of safety by the methods used for orthodox drugs; the herbalists, on the other hand, deeming current scientific methodology very crude and inadequate for measuring the fuller effects of the herb (and if the role of the practitioner, individual response, patient enrolment – in short, all the trappings of the paradigm – are

included, measurement becomes practically impossible). In 1982
the herbalists could say:

> It seems scarcely credible that a series of laboratory experiments
> over a few years could be so readily accepted against the use of
> a herbal remedy that has been taken for centuries in many
> areas of the world. (NIMH 1982: 1)

There is still greater pressure today to 'prove' herbs are safe and
more protestations by orthodoxy that tradition alone is inadequate
and far from rigorous enough to appease consumer concern and compare favourably with the rigour of orthodox drug testing. While herbalists are undoubtedly influenced by such exhortations and are being
obliged to make some moves in the orthodox direction, tradition
nevertheless still plays an important role in the ethos of their work –
a tradition based on a view of nature as greater than can be encompassed by rationality. Yet one can question too whether tradition and
ritual are not part of scientists' ethos. On this point Wynne develops
Kuhn's work on tradition and dogma in scientific research:

> Their consensus-maintaining power rests upon the socialised
> faith in the guidance of scientific belief by utterly impersonal
> rational rules. This too is a social ritual by which professions
> gain and maintain their social credibility and security. (Wynne
> 1976: 337)

For orthodox scientists, laboratory experiments lead to universal
knowledge; they are accessing the 'pure' effects of a substance on
the body. For the alternative camp the context is all important.
Even when they are not questioning the rigour of the laboratory
findings, they are questioning their relevance.

In the comfrey debate the question of why the laboratory results
should be taken seriously is an institutional, cultural and paradigmatic one and may be restated as what are the relations of power and
the respective interests of the relevant actors such that laboratory
findings appear more 'true' than other types of data? Shapin (1979),
in his paper on the professional anatomists' conflict with the phre-
nologists in the phrenology debate, suggests that social conflict and
ideological considerations may be seen as an important element in
the development of bodies of knowledge valued as 'interest free'.

All other experiments reporting toxicity of comfrey on laboratory
animals have been based on intraperitoneal injections of isolated
alkaloids – with the exception of those by Hirono. Hirono *et al.*

(1978) in Japan carried out an experiment in which the whole plant comfrey was used. Three groups of 19–28 inbred rats each were fed comfrey leaves for 480 to 600 days; four additional groups of 15–24 rats were fed comfrey root for varying lengths of time. Liver tumours were found in all groups except the controls, when autopsied at death.

Bone (n.d.) and Pembery (1982) again criticize the paper. PA levels were never measured, toxicity was admitted to vary. Diets of comfrey at certain levels are protein deficient and the effect of PAs is accentuated in protein deficiency. Six hundred days is a long time in the life of a laboratory rat; according to Pembery (1982) 80 per cent on a basal diet survive sixty days. The comparative control group survival was not indicated. Pembery again extrapolated figures and argues that the average rat consumed twenty-four times its own body weight at which level only one rat showed toxic symptoms. Bone's (n.d.) main criticism of the paper is the misleading nature of the title 'Carcinogenic activity of Symphytum officinale'. Symphytum officinale is referred to as Russian comfrey in the text, so it is unclear which comfrey is on trial (Upplandicum being reputedly far more toxic than officinale due to the combination of alkaloids found in it). But, more importantly, the tumours in all but three of the rats were benign; they were hepatotoxic, but not carcinogenic. Metastases were not mentioned, indicating the three cancerous tumours were of low malignancy. Malignancy occurred in the lower dosage groups, therefore a dose-response relationship was not evident. Yet this paper is cited frequently in subsequent reports as concrete evidence of carcinogenic properties of comfrey in animals.

There is no evidence of carcinogenic activity in humans. It is interesting to note that in Jamaica where incidence of liver lesions is high, cases of liver cancer are rare. Other reports on comfrey fed directly to animals report only favourable effects.

Evidence of Toxicity in Humans

The most often cited paper demonstrating toxicity of PAs in humans is that of Mohabbat *et al.* (1976), describing an outbreak of veno-occlusive disease in Afghanistan after contamination of wheat by Heliotropium seeds. Bone (n.d.) again criticizes the paper in that of two estimates of PA content the authors chose a lower one which would demonstrate chronic poisoning rather than acute, and enumerates anomalies in the choice of the lower figure, such as the impossibility of detecting PAs in urine at the lower intake rate. He suggests this case was again complicated by malnutrition, when toxicity is enhanced.

Coltsfoot has been banned in Germany as another plant containing PAs. Coltsfoot was identified as the active ingredient in a herbal tea mixture consumed by a pregnant woman during pregnancy, which led to the death of the baby from veno-occlusive disease at twenty-seven days old. Bergner (1990) records that although coltsfoot appeared on the label of the tea, the PA of coltsfoot, senkirkine, was not present. Senecionine had been isolated, a PA found in Petasites species, and a possible adulterant of coltsfoot. The mother acknowledged occasional consumption of cannabis and hallucinogenic mushrooms, though her liver was undamaged. Coltsfoot (or Petasites) formed only 9 per cent of the tea mixture. It was nevertheless banned as a result of this case.

Before the mid-1980s the defenders of comfrey were able to assert that no cases of comfrey poisoning had ever been discovered. But since then four cases have come to light which are the focus of renewed attempts at banning the herb. Yet again none of the cases is uncomplicated.

Case 1 (Ridker *et al.* 1985) A forty-nine-year-old woman was admitted to hospital with progressive swelling of the abdomen and extremities over the preceding four months. Veno-occlusive (v-o) disease was eventually diagnosed, allegedly caused by chronic exposure to PAs consumed in a comfrey powder, estimated at a minimum of 85mg of PAs over the previous six-month period. There were other possible causes of her illness; she was a heavy consumer of herbs, vitamins and 'natural' food supplements. These included daily supplementations of vitamins C, K, E, A, and B complex, calcium, magnesium, potassium, zinc, iron, lecithin and stereotrophic adrenal bovine extract. She drank three cups of chamomile tea per week, and for the six months before admission had consumed one quart per day of a herbal tea known as Mu-16. In addition, for the four months before admission, she had taken two capsules of 'comfrey-pepsin pills' with each meal. Only the Mu-16 tea and comfrey were considered as the harmful agents and despite admitting 'the total pyrrolizidine consumption we can establish for this patient is relatively low. It is possible that she had other sources of exposure and it is probable that she had been consuming pyrrolizidine containing supplements for longer than the period we could establish', the authors nevertheless conclude: 'To our knowledge, this is the first report of v-o disease in any human

after the use of a preparation claiming to be made from comfrey'
(Ridker *et al*. 1985: 1053). The title of the paper reads: 'Hepatic
veno-occlusive disease associated with consumption of PA-containing dietary supplements'.

Case 2 (Weston *et al*. 1987) A thirteen-year-old boy was admitted
into hospital with symptoms which were found to be caused by v-o
disease. He had been suffering from Crohn's disease for three years
and had been treated with prednisolone and sulphasalazine which
removed symptoms. At his parents' request the drugs were discontin-
ued and he was treated with acupuncture and comfrey root prescribed
by a naturopath. Exact quantities and frequency are unknown. He
had a further course of prednisolone in 1984. When admitted to
hospital he was taking prednisolone and sulphasalazine. The authors
point out that major hepatic vein thrombosis, but not v-o disease,
has been described in patients with colitis; they concede that the
patient may have been more susceptible to hepatic v-o disease because of underlying bowel disease causing malnutrition, but they
conclude that 'the only possible causal factor in this patient was
comfrey'. The drugs are not considered. The paper was entitled
'Veno-occlusive disease of the liver secondary to ingestion of comfrey'
(Weston *et al*. 1987: 183).

Case 3 (Bach *et al*. 1989) A forty-seven-year-old white non-alcoholic
woman began to feel unwell in 1978 with vague abdominal pain,
fatigue and allergies. A homoeopathic doctor recommended comfrey
tea. She consumed as many as ten cups per day in addition to taking
comfrey pills by the handful, which continued for more than one
year. Four years later, in 1982, serum aminotransferase levels were
twice the normal range. By 1986 she had further signs of liver disease. In this case it is not clear what the woman first presented with,
nor how long before the liver abnormalities developed she stopped
taking comfrey. In a case of addiction such as this, deleterious effects
are still counted as condemning the plant taken in normal, moderate
doses. The title of this paper was unambiguous: 'Comfrey herb tea-
induced hepatic veno-occlusive disease'.

Case 4   (Yeong *et al*. 1990) A twenty-three-year-old man presented with v-o disease and severe portal hypertension, and subsequently died from liver failure. He had eaten comfrey leaves for
some time before his illness. The man presented with a three-
month history of initial influenza-like symptoms followed by continued malaise and night sweats. Three weeks before admission

he noticed peripheral oedema and abdominal distension. For four years prior to illness he had been living on a commune and ate a predominantly vegetarian diet. He had a striking 'binge-type' eating pattern whereby he would eat large quantities of a particular food such as grapes or cashews for days and weeks on end. In the one to two weeks before the onset of symptoms he ate four to five steamed young comfrey leaves as a vegetable every day. The conclusion again is poisoning by comfrey. The details of the case are not clear – he ingested comfrey one to two weeks before onset of symptoms, but which symptoms – the initial flu-like ones three months previously or the more recent oedema and distension? The author suggests that the patient's protein deficient diet could have played a contributory role and admits that 'marked individual variations in dosage susceptibility have been found with other PAs'. Again the title implies certainty: 'Hepatic veno-occlusive disease associated with comfrey ingestion'.

None of the above cases is uncomplicated, each involves either abuse or other sources of toxicity. The link to comfrey cannot be made without considerable qualification.

The claim is now being made that ingestion of comfrey will show up as toxic perhaps a long time after consumption has stopped. Such a claim is almost impossible to prove or disprove.

Strategies

These are just a few examples of the complex nature of the debate. Throughout the literature strategies on the part of orthodoxy to marginalize comfrey can be detected.

Uncertainty exists at every stage of the process, yet in the reports the uncertainty is mostly ignored: the levels of PAs in the leaves or roots is never the same in any two experiments; indeed never the same in any two leaves. The young leaves have a higher level, the mature ones lower; levels in the leaves vary seasonally, being higher in spring. The nature of the alkaloids in the plants is not firmly established, for example there is doubt whether echimidine appears in Symphytum officinale or not. The effects on different laboratory animals differ: according to Pembery (1982) the LD50 (the dosage at which 50 per cent of the animals die) of retrosine in male rats is about 40mg/kg body weight, whereas guinea pigs had no liver damage at 420mg/kg.

The preparation of comfrey for use in experiments is taken as unproblematic. Yeong describes his preparations:

1.5kg of fresh roots and leaves of the hybrid Symphytum x upplandicum Nyman were freeze-dried and chopped. The plants were authenticated by the Botany Division, Department of Scientific and Industrial Research. The plant material was extracted exhaustively with methanol and the filtered extract was reduced in volume. The precipitated allantoin was filtered off and the methanol removed in vacu. The residue was dissolved in acid, washed with hexane and ether, treated with zinc dust to reduce the N-oxides, made alkaline and extracted with chloroform ... eighteen inbred dark Aguti rats aged 3–3 and half months were used ... the rats in group 1 were each fed by gavage, a single dose of 200mg/kg alkaloid dissolved in 3ml of 0.1M hydrochloric acid as the alkaloid is only partially soluble in water ... the livers (after sacrifice) were fixed in 10% formal saline ... sections were stained with hematoxylin and eosin and Gordon and Sweet's reticulin stain ... tissue from each liver was fixed in half strength Karnovsky's fixative, embedded in Epon 812 and examined .... (Yeong *et al.* 1991: 36)

Dolby (1979), talking about orthodox and deviant science, says 'each orthodox scientist builds upon apparent consensus and his original contributions offer arguments which extend it further' (Dolby 1979: 14). There is evidence of this in the comfrey literature. All papers after Hirono *et al.* (1978) (rats fed on comfrey for 600 days) which consider comfrey toxicity quote Hirono as having 'proven' the carcinogenicity of comfrey. Most quote Mohabbat *et al.* (1976) and Culvenor *et al.* (1980) both of which are flawed according to Bone (n.d.) and Pembery (1982). In particular, Winship (1991) (Medicines Control Agency), the papers by Ridker (McDermott and Ridker 1990; Ridker *et al.* 1985) (all based upon one case history from 1984), two by Yeong *et al.* (1990; 1991) and the Lawrencian Review (1987) are important papers based on these reports.

Dolby (1979) further says, 'scientists often ignore work with which they disagree, rather than openly challenge it' (Dolby 1979: 13). An example of this strategy can be found in the comfrey case: After the warning published in 1978 by Hills in the *BMJ* for the Doubleday Institute, investigations were made and the report by Pembery was subsequently published in 1982 in which the 1978 report was revoked and comfrey declared safe. Many of the papers after 1982 quote the 1978 warning and ignore the 1982 revocation; none cites the 1982 version. Statements in both Yeong *et al.* (1991) and Culvenor *et al.* (1980) which do refer to the unclear nature of the problem are rarely quoted in the subsequent literature. For example:

the safety of comfrey cannot be adequately gauged from existing data, although concern continues to be expressed regarding its usage. For a herb that is taken world-wide, only three cases of human hepatotoxicity have been reported. It is likely that the majority of consumers take the herb ... with impunity ... In a sample of dried comfrey leaves purchased from a local store, we found no evidence of PA. (Culvenor *et al.* 1980: 378)

Rather, the apparently more damning evidence is cited.

Imprecision, despite the scientific nature of the papers, abounds. Yeong describes his later work on rats: 'Three groups of young adult rats were fed PAs derived from Russian comfrey to study the effects *of the herb* on the liver' (Yeong *et al.* 1991: 35; emphasis added). Again the assumption stands that the PAs are an accurate measure of the whole plant. McDermott and Ridker (1990) present a very sketchy case history of their patient in their 1990 paper, omitting much information that would change the bias of the case: 'further review of the clinical history revealed that the patient had patronised health food stores for some years and had consumed large amounts of comfrey tea' (McDermott and Ridker 1990: 525). Compare this with the fuller case history above (Case 1).

Orthodox Cases

If we examine similar circumstances involving orthodox drugs, the arguments used to condemn comfrey, such as reaction to above normal doses, use of tradition, possible long-term toxicity and so on, do not apply.

In an exchange of letters in the *American Journal of Medicine* (Gumaste 1989), right beside a letter from Ridker on comfrey toxicity, two cases of acute pancreatitis induced by erythromycin are discussed. While the differences between the cases are outlined, their common feature appears to account adequately for the anomaly of the reaction: 'Both cases occurred as a result of above-normal doses ... Therefore, as suggested in my report, acute pancreatitis is probably an adverse effect encountered only with above-normal doses' (Gumaste 1989: 701); that is, abuse is tolerated, the drug is not under threat.

Herbalists are castigated for their reliance on tradition as proof of safety of their remedies. In a paper by Larrey *et al.* (1992), discussing cases of hepatitis after Germander administration, case 3 was a man who had taken Germander to lose weight and who was also taking dexfenfluramine. The authors do not rule out the latter as a cause of the man's hepatitis, but suggest that 'this drug has been marketed for several years and has not been reported to be hepatotoxic' (Larrey *et al*. 1992: 130). In other words 'tradition' can be mobilized rhetorically to defend orthodox drugs.

Another example concerns a paper in which the authors accept the use of metronidazole which was continued indefinitely in a patient with inflammation of an ileostomy despite the possibility that long-term use might be carcinogenic as indicated by tests on laboratory rats (McCleod *et al*. 1986).

Admittedly dangerous side-effects are of little consequence in the regulating and prescribing of orthodox drugs. For example, the *Independent* of 9 September 1992 reported that about 30,000 people are admitted to hospital each year with bleeding ulcers and about 3000 of them die. Between 20 and 30 per cent of the fatalities are caused by Non Steroidal Anti-inflammatory Drugs. GPs are aware of the risks but there has been no reduction in the 24 million prescriptions written.

It is interesting to note, in the context of the comfrey controversy, a comment of Professor Smith of the Institute of Environment and Health, in response to a 1995 report linking chemicals in the environment to falling sperm count in humans, reported in the *Guardian*:

> Just because a certain chemical tried out on rats in a lab causes them to get cancer in the testicles, it does not mean that tiny doses in the environment have the same effect on man and it should be banned. We are not in the business of making the world safer for rats to live in. (Brown 1995)

As noted above, the threat to comfrey now rests with the EU. Comfrey is on the list of the Committee for Proprietary Medicinal Products (CPMP) as one of the plants banned in one or more member states as possessing risks but of no proven benefit. The CPMP will decide in the future whether to make the ban Europe-wide.

Conclusion

This chapter reflects the mobilizing of orthodoxy against the challenge from alternative medicine. The science upon which the case against comfrey is based has not been carried out within the scientific frame of reference; it is not 'rigorous science' but lends itself rather to an interpretation as normative rhetoric. In a debate where uncertainty abounds, parameters are portrayed as certain. Even where uncertainty is acknowledged, scientific opinion prevails – for example, the Committee on Toxicity (COT) report on comfrey reads:

> We recognise that the four case reports of human veno-occlusive disease are isolated and anecdotal and we cannot be completely certain of a causal link with comfrey ingestion. Nevertheless veno-occlusive disease is a rare condition and is often associated with the consumption of plants and seeds containing PAs. Thus we consider it probable that comfrey products were implicated in these cases. (COT 1993: 1)

Through the power of the orthodox profession, supported by claims to access to truth through the rigour of their science, orthodox attacks on comfrey have been effective, despite charges of irrationality. The alternative camp remains relatively powerless in their defence of an alternative world-view and their challenge of normative science goes effectively unnoticed.

The comfrey controversy represents a clash of paradigms in Kuhnian terms, and highlights the incommensurability of one paradigm in terms of the other. In this case a reductionist yardstick which isolates chemicals from whole plants, tests them on animals and extrapolates to humans, following procedure for orthodox drugs with one basic action for use on a passive patient, proves inadequate and inappropriate for measuring a process where interrelationships, on a micro (plant) and macro (patient/practitioner) scale, are a fundamental tenet of the approach.

Wynne's work on Barkla can again be cited appropriately. He concludes:

> Scientists, we thought, were guided by objective, impersonal rules – they could hence offer to society, certainty. Commitment followed from the impersonal attainment of truth. However, in science, too, we now see social actors committing themselves in, and being committed by, historically developed situations, in circumstances of ultimate uncertainty and ambivalence. We should not be surprised if, like others, scientists attempt to reduce the personal and social tensions and insecurities of such circumstances by painting black and white over what is grey. But neither should we be awed into accepting the result at face value. (Wynne 1976: 338)

Herbalists do have a duty to ensure their herbs are safe. It makes more sense, however, for this investigation to proceed in terms of their own paradigm, and this need not be woolly and unfocused – there is no excuse for 'sloppy' practice in any paradigm. Attention needs to be focused on the plant in context, the synergistic action both of its own constituents and in conjunction with other remedies, and the action in individual patients in a therapeutic context. This then gives a more accurate reflection of the plant as therapeutic agent.

The debate about comfrey has concentrated here only on the safety aspect. The equally contentious issue of efficacy implicates the same consideration of paradigmatic demands and is relevant to complementary medicine as a whole. Given that recovery from illness depends on active patient involvement, then the subjective experience offers valuable information that forms an essential part of the interaction. The construction of the individual and society implicit in the paradigm demands a recognizing of context, of the collaborative generation of knowledge and of the relevance of 'non-scientific' expertise. The challenge is, then, as is happening in the environmental arena, to develop a science that admits uncertainty, that acknowledges the contribution of other dimensions of experience and represents a 'science in context'.

References

Bach, N. et al. (1989) 'Comfrey Herb Tea-induced Hepatic Veno-occlusive Disease'. American Journal of Medicine 87 97–9.
Barnes, B. (1982) T. S. Kuhn and Social Science. London: Macmillan.
Bergner, P. (1990) 'Comfrey, Coltsfoot and Pyrrolizidine Alkaloids'. Townsend Letter for Doctors. Feb/March.
Bone, K. (n.d.) Studies in Materia Medica Part 1 Symphytum Species. Tunbridge Wells: School of Herbal Medicine.
British Herbal Medicine Association (1985) British Herbal Pharmacopoeia 202–3.
British Medical Journal (1979) Unauthored statement. March 1979, 6163: 598.
Brown, Paul (1995) Guardian, 26 July, p. 5.
Committee on Toxicity (1993) Statement on the Safety-in-use of Comfrey.
Culpepper, N. (1979 reprint) Complete Herbal. Hong Kong: Gareth Powell.
Culvenor, C. et al. (1980) 'Structure and Toxicity of the Alkaloids of Russian Comfrey, a Medicinal Herb and Item of Human Diet'. Experientia 36: 377–9.

Dolby, R. (1979) 'Reflections on Deviant Science', in R. Wallis, *On the Margins of Science: The Social Construction of Rejected Knowledge*. Sociological Review Monograph. Staffs: University of Keele.

Gumaste, V. (1989) Acute Pancreatitis Induced by Erythromycin: The Reply. *American Journal of Medicine* 87: 701.

Hirono et al. (1978) 'Carcinogenic Activity of Symphytum Officinale', *Journal of National Cancer Institute* 61(3): 469–71.

Jago, M. (1971) 'Factors Affecting the Chronic Hepatotoxicity of Pyrrolizidine Alkaloids'. *Journal of Pathology* 105: 1–11.

Kuhn T. S. (1970) *The Structure of Scientific Revolutions*. Chicago: University of Chicago Press, 2nd edition.

Kumana, C. et al. (1985) 'Herbal Tea Induced Veno-occlusive Disease: Quantification of Toxic Alkaloid Exposure in Adults'. *Gut* 26: 101–4.

Larrey, D. et al. (1992) Hepatitis After Germander (Teucrium Chamaedrys) Administration: Another Instance of Herbal Medicine Hepatotoxicity. *Annals of Internal Medicine* 117(2): 129–32 (p. 131).

Lawrencian Review of Natural Products (1987) *Comfrey*. Pennsylvania: Pharmaceutical Information Associates.

McCleod, R. et al. (1986) 'Single Patient Randomised Clinical Trial'. *Lancet* 1: 1726–8.

McDermott, W. and Ridker, P. (1990) 'The Budd-Chiari Syndrome and Hepatic Veno-occlusive Disease, Recognition and Treatment'. *Archives of Surgery* 4(125): 525–7.

McIntyre, M. (1988) 'Comfrey', in R. Mabey, *The Complete New Herbal*. London: Elm Tree Books, p. 33.

McIntyre, M. (1995) *Herbs for Migraine*. Address given at Conference of National Institute of Medical Herbalists, Cirencester, April 1995.

Mills, S. (1991) *Out of the Earth, the Essential Book of Herbal Medicine*. London: Viking.

Mohabbat et al. (1976) 'An Outbreak of Hepatic Veno-occlusive Disease in NW Afghanistan'. *Lancet* 2: 269–71.

Mulkay, M. (1972) *The Social Process of Innovation: a Study in the Sociology of Science*. London: Macmillan.

National Institute of Medical Herbalists (1982) *Comfrey as a Medicine*. Press release.

Pembery, J. (1982) *The Safety of Comfrey*. Special report by the Henry Doubleday Research Association, Essex.

Ridker, P. et al. (1985) 'Hepatic Veno-occlusive Disease Associated with Consumption of PA-containing Dietary Supplements'. *Gastroenterology* 88: 1050–4.

Shapin, S. (1979) 'The Politics of Observation: Cerebral Anatomy and Social Interests in the Edinburgh Phrenology Disputes', in R. Wallis (ed.) *On the Margins of Science: The Social Construction of Rejected Knowledge*. Sociological Review Monograph, Staffs: University of Keele.

Weston, C. et al. (1987) 'Veno-occlusive Disease of the Liver Secondary to Ingestion of Comfrey'. *British Medical Journal* 295: 183.

Whitelegg, M. (1995) 'An Alternative Science for Herbal Medicine'. *European Journal of Herbal Medicine* 2(1): 36–9.

Winship, K. (1991) 'Toxicity of Comfrey'. *Toxicology Review* 10(1): 47–59.

Wynne, B. (1976) 'C. G. Barkla and the J. Phenomenon – A Case Study in the Treatment of Deviance in Physics'. *Social Studies of Science* 6: 307–47; (p. 337).

Yeong, M. *et al.* (1990) 'Hepatic Veno-occlusive Disease Associated with Comfrey Ingestion'. *Journal of Gastroenterology and Hepatology* 5: 211–14.

Yeong, M. *et al.* (1991) 'The Effects of Comfrey Derived PAs on Rat Liver'. *Pathology* 1(23): 35–8.

PART TWO

The Social Construction of Knowledge in Practice

Knowledge does not exist simply in a codified and written form. On the contrary, knowledge is embedded in professional practices; in communication between the practitioner and patient; in tacit, unarticulated decision making by the practitioners; in the material practices of the consulting room; and not least in the experiences of the patient. In this section the various locations of knowledge are explored. There is particular emphasis upon the relationship between codified and uncodifed knowledge and attention is turned to the ways in which knowledge is produced and communicated.

Richenda Power reflectively examines her role as a practitioner and the ways in which she notes information about patients and in doing so produces a knowledge resource. Ethical dilemmas are also discussed, in particular, how should the knowledge of individual patients be classified, stored and used? She asks who owns this knowledge – does it rightly belong to the patient? But, if so, how can such rich data be ignored and not appropriated for research and analysis?

Helle Johannessen's discussion of the patient–practitioner encounter illustrates that knowledge exists in a separate and additional form to that found in the textbook. The holistic premise that patients be treated individually and the fact that practitioners all have their own individual therapeutic preferences and prejudices combine to produce a situation where decisions about treatments are the product of intuitive negotiation. This implicit process rests alongside the deployment of more explicitly structured and codified knowledge about particular remedies and treatment regimes.

All knowledge of course has unstandardized dimensions, is imbued with values and interpretation, but these two chapters collectively illustrate how such knowledge comes to be constructed and used in practice. This uncodified aspect of the knowledge does not mean that it is *ad hoc* or marginal; implicit processes are central to the decision making involved in therapeutic encounters, whether in the complementary or the orthodox clinic.

4 Considering Archival Research in One's Own Practice

Richenda Power

A cluster of factors brought me to the point of considering archival research. Pressure for space in one clinic meant having just one tall filing cabinet, which became so tightly packed that files occasionally 'disappeared': some 'weeding out' seemed necessary. My method was to remove the files of people seen once more than five years previously, and of those I knew to have moved or died. I could not bring myself to destroy these potentially valuable sources of material for research so I stored them safely for future reference.

Celebrating ten years in practice in 1993 encouraged a 'taking stock', developed further by several events and meetings. A number of UK osteopaths, initially concerned to address the ethics of conducting research in practice, started discussion that year, becoming the Enabling Group for Osteopathic Research (EGOR), meeting regularly to encourage would-be osteopathic researchers.

Previously, Margaret Stacey, whose work on accountability in health care practice is well known (Stacey 1991; 1992; 1994), had directed me towards the group Consumers for Ethics in Research (CERES). CERES is unusual in its commitment to the research subjects' point of view. In the termly public meetings it is very powerful to hear research subjects speaking alongside researchers. For example, Anya Souza, who has Down's syndrome, spoke at a meeting on research in antenatal screening; and at a meeting devoted to research in psychiatry Rosalind Caplin, a mental health survivor, spoke alongside Dr Jim Birley, a psychiatrist. What hits one sharply in these juxtapositions are the differences between the speakers' perspectives on what is urgent and important for research; of what is acceptable or unacceptable as research practice and procedure.

In 1994, studying 'Professional Judgement and Decision-Making' (Open University 1992) helped structure my ideas further. This course uses medicine as illustration but its content is applicable to any situation where judgements are made about individual cases. For project work I reviewed my case-history recording practices. That is the background to this chapter. Earlier, shared as 'work in progress' (30 April 1994, Keele) I presented it as two main areas of interest, for clinical practice and education, and for sociology, commenting that this was a somewhat artificial separation. Sections on these two areas are preceded by two discussions: first, some ethical issues arising from the use of health records; and, second, of answers to a range of questions a social historian might put to any archive to establish its status. Applications relevant to both clinical feedback and sociological research are discussed in turn and finally drawn together with reference to articulating 'the relations between theory and practice, and also between language and the body' (Bourdieu 1990: 166). This is not a guide to conducting archival research but represents a process of thinking about it.

Ethical Issues

Clinical records should be kept securely so that only those who need to know their contents for health care reasons have access to them. The underlying assumption is that confidentiality should be maintained, which links to a belief in the sacrosanct privacy of an individual, whether patient or practitioner, lay or expert. This notion is common to many areas of work and says something about social attitudes to the individual and the relationship between the public and the private at interfaces such as practitioner–patient. Whilst much profession-produced literature makes claims to safeguarding confidentiality for its lay users it seems lay views are seldom publicly expressed on the matter. In addition it is still hard for patients to gain access to their notes despite legislation in Britain enabling this. Whether one's notes have been or may be used for research without one's knowledge or consent is another issue that intertwines with that of confidentiality.

The 'Ownership' of Records and Consent

In the British National Health Service, standard forms bear a message such as: 'THIS RECORD IS THE PROPERTY OF THE SECRETARY OF STATE FOR HEALTH'. Guidelines apply to the minimum length of time records should be kept (UK Department of Health Circular 1989), but as yet these do not apply to 'unofficial' (Larner's term,

1984) practitioners in private practice. Some implications of this ownership were spelt out by Dr Birley, saying that much research was not done face to face but 'on people's notes' (Birley 1994). My thoughts were that patients consult for help with their health, not to be unwitting research subjects with consent implicit in the encounter when notes are made.

Such 'consent' appears to be assumed by the Medical Research Council (MRC) and the Royal College of Physicians (RCP), which presents the MRC's statement as authority:

> it would not be practicable to seek the consent of each and every patient. Sometimes many thousands of records are involved. Frequently, records must be included on patients who are unavailable or untraceable because of changes of abode, migration or death. In some research, obtaining consent in itself may cause needless anxiety. The Council therefore consider that, subject to scrupulous safeguards about confidentiality, information about patients can properly be available for medical research without their explicit consent, as it has been in the past. (MRC statement quoted in RCP 1990b: 13)

Despite this 'official' line, Birley argued that consent is an ongoing issue, not a one-off event, backing this up with evidence of differences between general practitioners' and patients' perceptions of information given at an encounter. One way to recognize and work with this is to give written information about the research to participants, to help them make informed decisions throughout the course of treatment.

Implications for the use of clinical records in future or for other purposes are not clear. An American social scientist, writing some time ago, held that:

> The analysis of information developed and assembled for reasons other than those of primary interest represents ... [an example] of *covert research*. Examples would be: the secondary analysis of research data that perhaps was originally collected with the knowledge, consent and co-operation of the participants .... (Reynolds 1982: 78; emphasis added)

For the patient such research on their health record might seem like prying into their private life, without their consent, possibly with damaging consequences. Reynolds (1982) stressed the need for researchers to demonstrate respect for participant rights and welfare, but the very word participant implies that the subject of research is aware of the fact of participating.

Priscilla Alderson of CERES commented that 'standards have changed very much in the last twenty years especially in medicine', and stressed ethical guidelines should 'be placed in the context of their time', as 'All ... are political statements with hidden agendas' (personal communication 1996).

Most British ethics committees' main concerns are to do with the nature of any procedures involved and their risk. 'Risk' could either be possible permanent damage or that involved in invasive procedures. The latter are 'often interpreted in a physical sense such that some research ethics committees dismiss talk as non-invasive' (Alderson, personal communication 1996). However, much research can be intrusive when asking people about their private and intimate lives. This is relevant for osteopathy, naturopathy and all 'holistic' therapy settings where case histories are taken.

I feel that only the practitioner and the patient should have access to the notes they jointly constructed, unless patients give their explicit consent to specific research. Issues of what the research is about, whose interests it is intended to serve, whether and where it may be published, who else might see one's personal material, and so on, must be addressed. The issue of confidentiality is intimately linked with these matters.

Confidentiality

An epidemiologist's stance might be that provided the information from notes is not identifiable and confidentiality is not breached then records can be used without concern about obtaining consent. Alderson points to the existence of a 'broad disagreement between clinicians (more pro-consent) and epidemiologists' (personal communication 1996). Clinical case studies carry an obvious risk of identification. For example, consider the study of rare situations, like Sachs's (1987) *The Man Who Mistook His Wife For A Hat* – so unusual it is identifiable. Similar concerns arise over books discussing psychoanalytic cases (for example, Pincus and Dare 1980), because, even where names are disguised, family circumstances, people's occupations and living arrangements are distinctive, and it is not possible to know, as a researcher, what harmful circumstances may arise from readers' access to this material. I speak from personal experience as an interviewee for a popular book, where, although my name was changed, there seemed to be sufficient detail for potential identification.

From experience of the impact of mental illness in my family, I was aware of the negative implications of having mental distress officially recorded and wanted to avoid being labelled. Consequently, when I had an 'eating disorder' I sought help from private sources, enjoying what I thought was an unusually confidential relationship, not accessible by the 'state'. It is possible that others consulting 'unofficial' practitioners do so precisely because they desire a privacy that the general practice or the hospital is unable to ensure.

Apart from the protection of individuals, specific minorities' rights should be considered. Confidentiality issues arise for people with rare genetic patterns who may well wish to hide from public gaze and state control, and also are concerned with the human immuno-deficiency virus (HIV). Reynolds discussed the issue of rare cases: 'extreme values may be omitted from tables (as the US Census Bureau does when the number of individuals represented is less than five)' (1982: 57).

Time is relevant too. For example, when someone dies from AIDS they, their family and friends may wish to keep this private, so any 'rule book' approach to records and research, for instance, that fifty years is sufficient protection (Zarzecka and Lorentzon 1995), could require revision. The UK census rule is 100 years. However, the importance of the availability of medical records for research is stressed by Homan (1991: 88–9), citing studies that established the link between smoking and lung cancer, an epidemiological point.

It seems clear that decisions about the length of time absolute confidentiality should be maintained are arbitrary, depending on historically and culturally mutable notions of potential damage to individuals and groups, and are often outweighed by professional power and research interests.

Reynolds summarized several techniques for maintaining anonymity: using code numbers and storing the identifying information separately; omitting rare cases;

eliminating the most salient information that might be used for identifying respondents; the microaggregation of data (such as summary descriptions of ten-person groups) or 'inoculation' (such as randomly modifying the ages by one or two years that would have a small effect on the analysis but would prevent positive identification of the respondents) ... (Reynolds 1982: 57)

but pointed out that 'maintaining anonymity is becoming a specialised technical area', referring to Boruch and Cecil (1979), as does Lee (1993: 14) more recently in a useful historical survey of 'research on sensitive topics'.

In addition to written records, pictures, sketches, photographs and diagrams are also present in case histories. Problems of identification are even more pressing here. Rosalind Caplin described the intrusion she experienced, aged fifteen, when she had to pose naked for photographs for an article in a medical journal. She felt she had not given consent, but was obliged to pose as demanded, alone with a male photographer. Her experience is illustrative of the potential abuse of patients, particularly children, by practitioners/ researchers (see Alderson 1995). Recent advice on the use of photographs is that the eyes need no longer be disguised if the patient has given full consent (*BMJ* 1995). However, should permission be obtained again if the picture is used for other publications, as it has to be from photographers and illustrators?

Records in my Practice

The records in my private practice do not belong to the state. However, they are concerned with personal material and therefore issues of confidentiality arise as well as the question of whether it is ethical to use a patient's notes for any purpose other than that for which they were originally constructed. Should I write to each patient and ask for their 'informed consent' to any research project I might do with their material? Perhaps not if I am purely reviewing records for my own private purposes, for instance looking at patterns of presentation, treatment and outcome to identify areas of strength and weakness in my practice.

If results are to be *published* in any sense, whether giving a talk to peers or having an article placed in a journal, then consent and confidentiality must be addressed. Their resolution should not depend ultimately upon some notion of the 'integrity' of the individual researcher and/or practitioner, nor on a set of professional guidelines that may be irrelevant to a particular context or fail to take the priorities of the research subjects into account. I have found it essential to my thinking to join in debates in settings such as CERES. There are no final or fixed answers.

As I was writing this chapter a few patients voiced extremely positive views on possible participation in research in osteopathy and naturopathy, suggesting I was over-concerned about consent and confidentiality. They felt anything that helped 'prove' the efficacy of such approaches, thereby helping 'recognition' and eventual inclusion in the British National Health Service had to be a 'good thing'. Such positive motivation should make practitioners/researchers even more careful about their ethical review.

Collaborative situations where, say, an osteopath is engaged at a state health centre, or a general practitioner formally refers a patient to a herbalist in a contractual arrangement, raise further issues to do with confidentiality and consent. Perhaps then the patient's notes do 'belong' to the state? The patient may wish to keep personal information compartmentalized between different practitioners, with implications for recording in the first place. Publishing research on collaborative settings can expose other practitioners so their consent should also be sought (see Harrison and Lyon 1993).

Overall the ethical issues arising from research on clinical records will be intimately linked with the purposes of that research. I move now to consider the status of clinical records as a resource.

Standard Social Historical Questions of Any Archive

When using documents for social research several questions that seek to establish their status must be addressed. Below I treat some of these standard issues in regard to my archive.

The initial construction of my clinical records is for health care, their primary purpose. Any research use to which they are put would be secondary. Apart from ethical questions already raised, issues to do with the problems of retrospection and recollection arise. I may interpret records differently from their original meaning, and thus reconstruct them. This is a standard problem for the social historian, from which the use of one's own material is not exempt.

Indeed, doing research in one's 'own field', particularly on one's own records, may have very specific problems to do with too much contextual material being taken for granted and not spelt out to the potential readers of the research, or neglected because it does not seem worthy of question. For example, it might be assumed that 'of course' every practitioner wanted to 'get the patient better', without attempting to specify exactly what that meant.

What are the records for? Gathered for the sake of the patient's health, they attempt to guide me through considering an appropriate diagnosis and treatment plan. Over time they record the review of that diagnosis and the progress or otherwise of the patient.

Increasingly they were written with communication in mind with people other than the patient: doctors to whom I might decide to refer, lawyers who might require my case notes for insurance claims and so on.

This leads to the question: Who is the audience? For myself, a record of observations made at a fixed point in time at first encounter; an awareness of the frame and the narrative that the patient presented; a record of my attempts to diagnose; and a record of my attempts to help produce change. The initial record is one against which I compare future observations. It may also be used for writing medical and legal reports with the authenticity of evidence gathered at the time.

I may write for a potential locum or another professional as a communication tool. The audience may be medical and that awareness may affect my choice of language, translating osteopathic concepts into the language of orthopaedics (as British osteopaths were advised to do for political reasons in the period approaching the Osteopaths' Bill, 1993). For a report I abstract conventional 'signs and symptoms' so that I speak the standard language of the medical profession.

For the patient, some may require to have their records. This could be particularly important as 'witness' work for those who have heard repeatedly that there is 'nothing wrong' when they have had many medical encounters and investigations (that is, a record as a potential political tool).

The record may also be a legal tool for me in the sense of a notation of what I thought I did or did not do, in the face of future litigation.

Further questions that may be raised regarding archival material are summarized by Webb *et al.* (1981: 163–4) in somewhat positivist vein (for example, questions to do with accuracy), and by Scott (1990) in a more interpretative framework. Theoretical 'traditions of documentary analysis' are concisely presented by Jupp and Norris (1993) as broadly positivist, interpretative or critical. The presentation of the rest of this chapter loosely follows that sequence of traditions, starting with a discussion of research for clinical feedback.

Archival Research for Clinical Feedback

A major purpose of the analysis of clinical records is epidemiological. Charting patterns of presentation, of prevalence of complaints in specified populations, of outcomes in different treatment conditions, can be used to answer some questions and to raise others. 'Clinical audit' has been required as part of an increasing emphasis on accountability since the British National Health Service reforms of April 1991 (see HMSO 1992) and this has influenced 'unofficial' medicine too (for example, Collins 1994). Distinctions are made between 'audit' and 'research' though this is the subject of much debate. A research proposal can be returned by one ethics committee marked 'this is audit, not research', whilst another decides that aspects of the same proposal are unethical, refusing access. The decision 'this is audit' implied that ethical approval was not required which tallies with the Royal College of Physicians' recommendation that

> Ethics Committees need not be concerned with work which involves what amounts to quality control, medical audit or preliminary clinical appraisal, including work to establish possible causes of disease .... (RCP 1990a: 22)

Such experiences illustrate the existence of a fuzzy boundary between 'audit' and 'research' which is debated in the medical press. It seems appropriate to consider and resolve ethical issues, whatever the label.

I shall now mention some of the simplest projects that could be designed using existing case-history records.

Possible Projects

In my case histories there is a category of presenting symptoms noted, followed by descriptions of an examination, with some sort of working diagnosis, maybe not spelt out explicitly, but implicit in the recorded treatment or referral decisions. Later perhaps an 'outcome' is recorded. In many 'unofficial' health care settings the 'diagnosis' may be more complex and perhaps more difficult to put into a one- or two-word label form than is usual in 'official' medicine.

Usually much more information is present. Often demographic details (age, address, sex, occupation) and doctor, previous treatments, family health history, and so on, are gathered. The main reason for consultation is noted along with other factors such as the quality of sleep, exercise, nutrition, life events and health history. I record progressively updated thoughts on diagnosis, observations of treatment outcome and revised decisions about prognosis.

One could access at any point of the multiple variables repeated across numerous case histories and look at various correlations. Several researchers have made such analyses of clinical records (for example, van der Toorn 1983; Berthon 1993). The only analysis I have completed so far (1985) is of my first 100 patients, when I received resounding criticism from senior naturopaths for taking too short-term and medical a view of 'cure'. The notion of measuring an 'outcome' when the view of health and illness is fundamentally different and symptoms are seen as 'friends' and part of a healing process is difficult to translate into a conventional medical audit model. (Although 'outcome' measurement is acknowledged to be challenging in medicine too (see Bowling 1991).)

In collaborative settings one's record keeping may be open to view by other professionals, and this may be mutual, so a variety of record-keeping practices and languages may be noticed. Britten's (1993) study of pharmacists' records highlighted their potential to observe patterns of prescribing by general practitioners. There may be mutual influence as language groups (for instance, osteopaths, general practitioners, aromatherapists) share documentation.

Considering such settings can encourage a shift from a purely positivist audit of archives towards a more interpretative framework that could look at competing and mutually influential discourses about the body. Whilst an actuarial approach to one's practice (Glaser 1985; Meehl 1986; Dawes 1988; Einhorn 1988) is important in terms of accountability, I am also fascinated by sociological research possibilities, some of which are discussed below.

Archives as Social Historical Resources

My research interests have been in both the sociology of knowledge and that of the professions (see Power 1991). This perhaps explains my interest in how people communicate from one 'body of knowledge' and practice to another. I consider all knowledge to be open to sociological investigation: mathematics and 'pure' sciences alongside more obviously 'applied sciences' like medicine (for example, see Wright and Treacher 1982), osteopathy and healing.

Here I outline some ideas that reflect on the construction of knowledge in clinical practice. If, as a sociologist, I analyse processes of construction of knowledge in other disciplines, I should be prepared to turn the analysis reflexively on my own process of knowledge construction, laying it bare. ('Reflexivity' is a major commitment of the 'strong programme'[1] in the sociology of knowledge.) This seems important also to my clinical work.

Below I describe some ways in which it could be possible, using archival records, to look first at the development of the practitioner over time, then at the practitioner as constructor of views of their patients. Finally, I consider comparative studies.

A Record of a Practitioner's Development

I can identify various professional developments that probably affected the way I practise, in terms of changes in what I examine, questions I ask and my diagnostic and treatment decisions. There was the starting point of graduation and beginning practice. I soon left my college's professional organization and joined another group of naturopaths with whom I felt more affinity. My whole approach to the patient felt shaken up by this because of fundamental disagreements about the philosophy of 'cure', and a stress on the avoidance of dependence by the patient on any factor other than 'nature' for healing (see Power 1994). When I became an external examiner for the General Council and Register of Osteopaths in 1990, I reappraised my clinical performance as I was obliged to assess others. Records following identified events could be sampled and examined for any changes that may have occurred. This systematic approach would enable an assessment of their effects.

Perhaps I could also measure the impact of common human experiences, which I hope have deepened my capacity for hearing what patients are saying, and for better appreciating the interplay between life events and bodily distress. (I think of experiences such as bereavement, litigation, housing and work insecurities.)

These are examples of the construction and reconstruction of the practitioner, traces of which might be found in the archive. Now I move to a discussion of the construction of the case history format itself.

The Record as a Construction: Picturing Bodies

At first I continued to use the case-history form on which I had been trained (Figure 4.1). Later I expanded the space for the 'patient's own story' and discarded the box 'mento-emotional habitus' which I felt was both inadequate as a space and also tended to push a practitioner toward a labelling approach ('hysteric', 'neurotic', 'balanced'?) which I

Figure 4.1 The case history on which I was trained.

BRITISH COLLEGE of NATUROPATHY & OSTEOPATHY

Practitioner

Ref. No. ....

Mr.
Mrs. .... (Married / Single) Age .... Occupation ....
Miss

Name ....

Address ....

Phone ....

Date ....

Chief Complaint: shoulder/upper △ strain

Present Illness: onset 1 mth ago - severe. but had noticed for previous 6 mths. pain ↑ in evening c. 5 p.m. absent in morning. worsens in evening. ↓ if lies on floor — stomach or back - flat on back best. pain - dull nagging creeps up → extreme tension: sometimes unbearable.
panic attacks: anxiety builds up. palpitations. hands shaking.
esp'y when alone + kids. c. 2x/week.

Past History:
0—10. UCD. 8 yrs. mumps + severe stiff painful neck afterwards. (not diag'). ?meningitis.
10 - 20 FMP 13. NAD.
20 → 21 1st child. pethidine. normal delivery. gluc. drip. longish labour. 18h. mild backache at base of back. towards end.
24. post both births backache much worse after labour.
noticed that backache returns in times of stress/shock etc.

Family History:

bowels: no problem. **PRESENT DIET AND LIVING HABITS** bladder: no problems

On rising

B'fast: sugar puffs/cornflakes, white toast ... butter, coffee

Mid-morning coffee.

Lunch: soup (tin) or sandwich. white bread. coffee

fresh fruit / apples. etc.

Afternoon:

Evening Meal: curry/fish + chips/roast dinner
brussels/peas/carrots (tinned)
onions/green peppers
fresh orange juice
salad 2x/week
white cabbage, mushrooms, tomatoes, cucumber. + vinegar + oil.

On retiring: coffee

pudding 2x/week
tinned fruit + apple
ice cream
crumble/custard

~~Tea:~~

Coffee: 5/day.

Alcohol: occ'.

Tobacco: 20/day.

Special Dietetic Factors: Rx: distalgesic. panadol. 2-3x/wk.
valium - has just stopped.
pyridoxine. 2x/day.

Sleep: wakes 1-3/night.
soft mattress.

Mento-Emot. Habitus:

Exercise: walking.

EXAMINATION

Tongue: NAD.	Nervous System:
Skin: NAD	
Cap. Circ. NAD	
Cardio-Vascular { Pulse NAD.	Eyes:
Heart	
B.P.	Ears:
Blood test NAD.	
Lungs & Resp:	Nose:
Abdomen:	Throat:
Genito-Urinary:	
	Extremities:

Structual Examination: C. 1b ↓ bilat ↑ ↓ ®

SIDE VIEW   BACK VIEW

CERVICAL
A
C
DORSAL   X tender (e lesion?)
B
LUMBAR
SACRAL   tender to palpate con movement
COCCYGEAL

		DATE							
URINALYSIS									
Colour	...								
Deposits	....								
pH.	...								
Sp. Grav.	...								
Albumen	...								
Sugar	...								
Blood	....								
Acetone	...								
Bilirubin	...								

Diagnosis:

Prognosis:

Summary of T'ment Advised:

PROGRESSIVE WEIGHT RECORD					
Date	Stones	Lbs.	Date	Stones	Lbs.

disliked. I incorporated more standard memory-joggers for ticking responses, partly because of time pressures but also because of a growing atmosphere in the UK of medico-legal accountability and the requirement for professionals to record everything tested, whether 'positive' or 'negative'. However, I continued to use the old picture (Figure 4.2). Some time later I dispensed with this to leave space for freehand drawing (Figures 4.3 and 4.4).

Figure 4.2   My first modification of the back page.

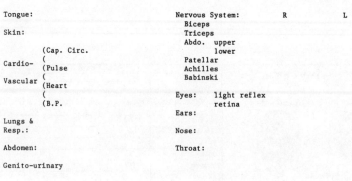

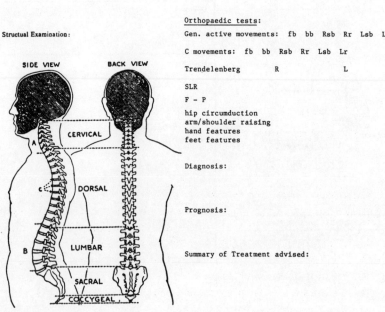

EXAMINATION

Tongue:

Skin:

Cardio- (Cap. Circ.
         (
Vascular (Pulse
         (
         (Heart
         (
         (B.P.

Lungs &
Resp.:

Abdomen:

Genito-urinary

Nervous System: R   L
  Biceps
  Triceps
  Abdo. upper
         lower
  Patellar
  Achilles
  Babinski

Eyes: light reflex
         retina
Ears:

Nose:

Throat:

Structual Examination:

SIDE VIEW   BACK VIEW

A   CERVICAL

C   DORSAL

B   LUMBAR

SACRAL

COCCYGEAL

Orthopaedic tests:

Gen. active movements: fb bb Rsb Rr Lsb Lr

C movements: fb bb Rsb Rr Lsb Lr

Trendelenberg   R   L

SLR
F - P

hip circumduction
arm/shoulder raising
hand features
feet features

Diagnosis:

Prognosis:

Summary of Treatment advised:

Figure 4.3 A later modification (c.1990).

Nose:			Skin:
smell			nails

Eyes:	R	L	Cardiovascular
visual fields			capillary On
pupillary reflex			pulse
retina			heart
trochlear			b.p.
abducens			

Respiration
rate

Ears:	expansion
hearing	fremitus
	percussion
Mouth:	auscultation
lips	
teeth	Abdomen
tongue	
gums	
	Genito-urinary
Throat:	
gag	

Nervous System

reflexes:	R	L	muscle tests:	R	L
biceps			shdrs (C34)		
triceps			Biceps (C56)		
br/rad			triceps (C78)		
abdo U					
abdo L			flexors		
patella			extensors		
Achilles			abductors		
Babinski			adductors		
			inversion		
			eversion		

Orthopaedic tests
Active movements
fb bb Rsb Lsb Rr Lr

Cervical movements
fb bb Rsb Lsb Rr Lr

	R	L
Tren/berg		
SLR		
F-P		
hip On		

arm raisg
hand features

feet features

DIAGNOSIS:

TREATMENT RECOMMENDED:

There were several reasons for doing this. Perhaps, first, it was a distaste for an ablist and conventional view of a straight spine. The prefix 'ortho-' – as in orthopaedics, orthodontics – means 'straight, rectangular, upright, correct' (Sykes 1982). The picture on which I trained was male: back and left side views, armless and legless. I enjoyed *A New View of a Woman's Body* (Federation of Feminist Women's Health Centers 1981), where Suzann Gage drew

Figure 4.4 Current format (1995).

```
name (contd)                date               page three
                         EXAMINATION
L view                    P view                A view
```

```
movements  fb  bb  Rsb  Lsb  Rr  Lr                    s-is
C
T                                                       LEX
L                                                       UEX

ENT:                                        DIAGNOSIS:

skin:
                                            PROGNOSIS:
CVS:
                                            TREATMENT GIVEN:

Resp:
                                            ADVICE GIVEN:

Abdo:

Genito-urinary:


Orthop. tests:



Neurol. tests:
```

real women in contrast to the diagrams of many gynaecological
texts. Her women are of various shapes, sizes, skin colours and
ages, and diagrams of wombs and ovaries are often contextualized
with illustrations of whole women instead of mere pelvic views.

Place (1993) discussed the construction of 'the visibility of a criti-
cally ill body' in the intensive care unit. He demonstrated a continuum of representation of the body from, say, a picture of a person

embedded in technology (that all would recognize) to that of the body as merely a small box in a flowchart diagram surrounded by machinery in the intensive care setting. His ideas encouraged me to try to 'bring bodies back in' as a political move towards information sharing with the patients (see changing representations of bodies on my case histories, Figures 4.5, 4.6 and 4.7).

Watching students I was struck by variations in terms of how long they spent on observation before examining the patient, and also whether they drew as they observed. There is a philosophical debate as to whether there is ever a possibility of 'authentic' or 'true' observation. Johnson Abercrombie, who taught zoology, referred to a problem:

When [the students were] asked to describe what they saw through the microscope, they often did not distinguish sufficiently sharply between what was there and what they had been taught 'ought' to be there. (Johnson Abercrombie 1989: 15)

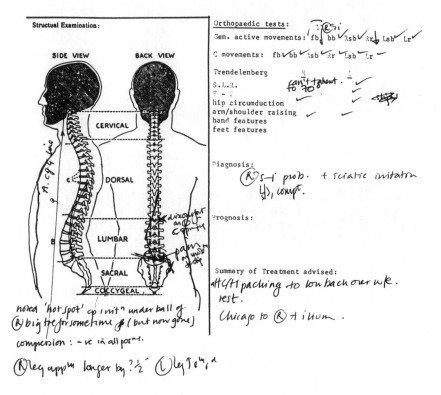

Figure 4.5 Example of the format in use.

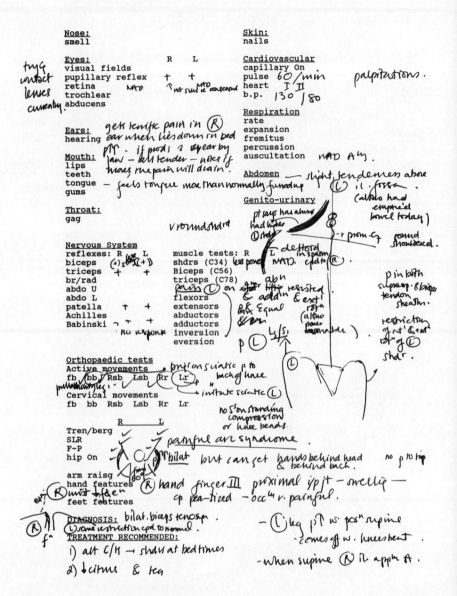

Figure 4.6 Example of the format in use.

Eric Sotto[2] discussed this text saying the student can be told where to look without being told what to see. But telling someone 'where to look' is problematic in itself in its assumption of the possibility of an 'authentic' or essential view. A view of the body

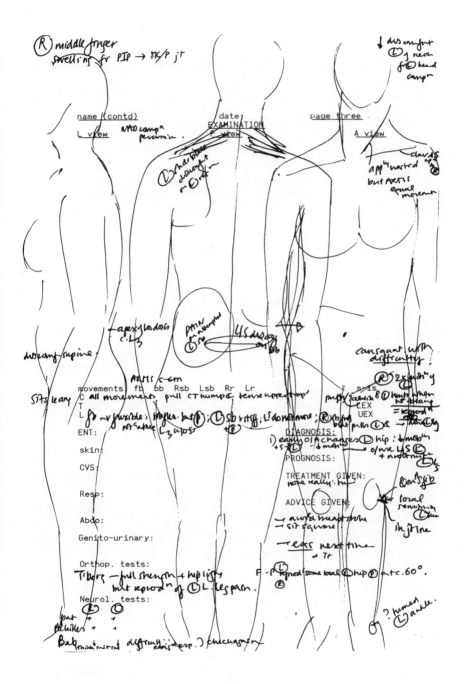

Figure 4.7 Example of the format in use.

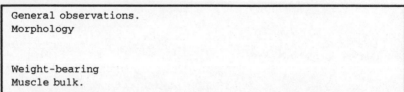

General observations.
Morphology

Weight-bearing
Muscle bulk.

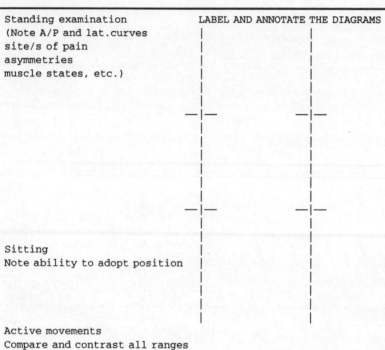

Standing examination   LABEL AND ANNOTATE THE DIAGRAMS
(Note A/P and lat.curves
site/s of pain
asymmetries
muscle states, etc.)

Sitting
Note ability to adopt position

Active movements
Compare and contrast all ranges

Figure 4.8 Part of the case-history format at the British School of Osteopathy, London (c. 1991).

seems always a trained view, whether that of a dancer, osteopath,
nurse, orthopaedic surgeon or mother.

In addition to the problem of visual perception and its frameworks, there is the challenge of creating two-dimensional records of
tactile perception. Those working 'hands on' (and perhaps 'hands off',
like some healers) may attempt to record sensations that as yet have
no shared encoding. There have been interesting debates about the
recording of levels of pain (Melzack and Wall 1982), and now, particularly in the cranial field of osteopathy, there are struggles to
express in language what is felt through hand and body.[3] Often I
found it easier to draw what I felt.

Case History Formats as Social Constructions

Above I described *my* development of record keeping. But I was a student for four years at a particular college. That training partly constructed my frame for viewing the patient. External examining elsewhere brought recording as *social* construction to my attention. The format favoured at any one college can be considered as the grid or the frame through which the patient starts to be perceived (see Figures 4.8 and 4.9). Some have legs and arms: does this make a difference to practice? Is the practitioner more likely to observe relationships say between the feet and the pelvis? The colleges' formats also change, moving from blank paper to the use of a full 'manne-quin' and back again.

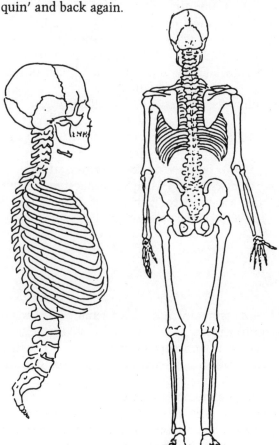

Figure 4.9   Part of a case-history format at the European School of Osteo-pathy, Maidstone, Kent (c. 1991).

Beyond comparative studies between colleges of osteopathy one could examine the ways other bodily disciplines have constructed methods and formats of notation. Take dance: to describe a way of holding the body, of moving the body, poses similar challenges to markmaking on the page, to codification. Neither video recording, photography nor virtual reality overcomes the construction of the frame.

Here debates about the relationship (if any) between representation and reality are pertinent (see Chaplin 1994 for a useful discussion). The record is produced from a particular way of observing selected cues. What counts as a cue varies from one convention of observing to another (see Gombrich 1977). Sally Macintyre (1978), who studied note making in an antenatal clinic, pointed out that it is not that there is a missed reality, but that the purposes of the note making and the frames of the note makers shape the nature of what gets recorded. This is not peculiar to clinical record making but, for example, in a conventionally 'basic science' for medicine – anatomy – Lord Zuckerman (1961: xi) wrote: 'No two anatomists are likely to agree precisely about what constitutes unnecessary detail in the dissecting room.' An examination of the range of anatomy textbooks quickly reveals a wide variety of emphases for different purposes (for example, see Lockhart 1948; Jepson 1960; McMinn and Hutchings 1990; Calais-Germain 1993). However, comparative studies of illustrations in these texts also enable us to raise questions about systematic patterns in the social space such as the dominance of bodies that are able to stand, that are male, and so on (see Mendelsohn et al. 1994).

An 'Artificial Separation'

Earlier I stated that I was using an 'artificial separation' between potential purposes of archival research, for sociology and for clinical practice and education. Here in summary I hope to weave together some of the threads I have drawn in considering uses of clinical archives.

Bourdieu highlighted sport and dance as areas

in which is posed with the maximum acuteness the problem of the relations between theory and practice, and also between language and the body. ... How can you make someone understand, that is, make someone's body understand, how he [sic] can correct the way he moves? The problems raised by the teaching of a bodily practice seem to me to involve a set of theoretical questions of the greatest importance, in so far as the social sciences endeavour to theorise the behaviour that occurs, in the greatest degree, outside the field of conscious awareness, that is learnt by a silent and practical communication, from body to body one might say. (Bourdieu 1990: 166)

Osteopathy, physiotherapy, chiropractic, shiatsu, and so on, all involve 'body to body' communication (see Figure 4.10 overleaf). What is objectified in clinical records is not the actual process of that communication but an attempt to record the unspoken agenda of change that both practitioner and patient negotiate.

The potential relevance the sort of archival research I suggest has for sociology and for clinical practice is in beginning to articulate something of the relations between theory and practice, and also between language and the body.

Clinical Feedback as Discourse

A person who presents their body to a health expert for treatment is usually pushed into action by the 'subjective' experience of pain, or an awareness of disturbance of function that was previously taken for granted (for example, being able to hold a kettle of water). The expert and the lay person may or may not share notions of the 'normal' experience of the body, whether it be an alignment of posture (taken for granted in diagrams of the skeleton in some case records), or of function as an autonomous independent being. These usually unspoken assumptions about bodies and their behaviour may be drawn out from case-history archives and demonstrate a structure of normative patterns of observing and using the body in different contexts. Such studies could explain why there are various systems of viewing the body which are differentially privileged in various social groups, cultural settings and even in whole societies.

Expectations of different class bodies have been remarked upon: the points at which people choose to engage with an expert's observation, instruction and manipulation (that is, to enter in a relationship via a specific frame) may vary across classes, gender, age, ethnicity, and so on (see Williams 1996). Archival studies may assist theoretical development in this regard.

The archival record is one-sided to the extent that it is formed by the expert. It is not a neutral observation of the interaction between

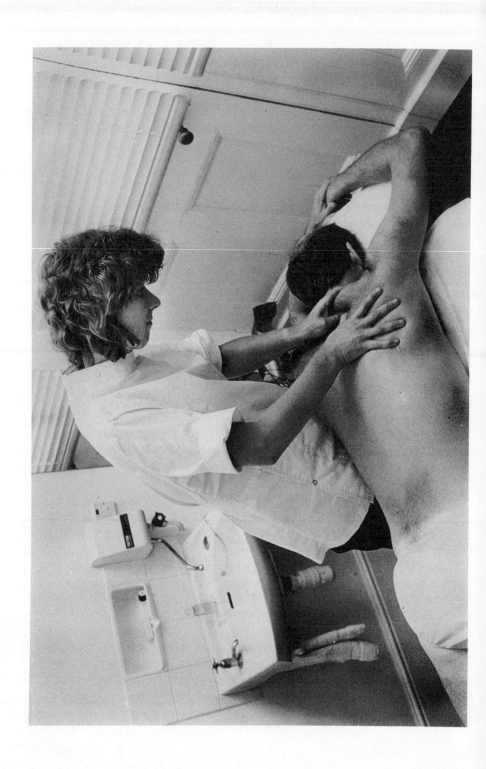

Figure 4.10 (opposite) Sanne van der Toorn, naturopath and osteopath, at work, 1985. © David Hoffman.

the practitioner and the patient. It is theoretically guided in its format, in the way in which the practitioner was trained to observe and to record. It is a snapshot in time, perhaps followed by subsequent snapshots. Underlying the construction of these is the agenda of the professional, the way a body is to be viewed, to be made to behave, to alter its behaviour. There is a micro-social analysis possible here of a power relationship. What is of interest to the social scientist and the clinician are the social patterns of encounters recorded in clinical records. As Cooter stressed, we may regard medical knowledge '... as a mediation of social experience, mutually constituted with it' (1982: 16). There is no getting away from this – even the study of anatomy is based on the dissection of cadavers of certain classes and possibly of particular ethnicities; only some bodies agree to this use or have no power to refuse. The presentation of the anatomically 'normal' is based on selected cases, whether living or dead. The practitioners who observe and manipulate the patients do not exist in isolation from the discourses of their particular period and setting. As I have shown above they may pick up the dominant and disagree with its use. In this way Bourdieu's words about sport, dance and music resonate with ideas about clinical practice with bodies.

A sport, at a given moment, is rather like a musical work: it is both the musical score (the rules of the game, etc.), and also the various competing interpretations (and a whole set of sedimented interpretations from the past); and each new interpreter is confronted by this, more unconsciously than consciously, when ... [she] proposes ... [her] interpretation. (Bourdieu 1990: 165)

In this sense the analysis of clinical records can lend itself also to a reading as autobiography. But that is a situated story and it is that interplay between the individuals (patient–practitioner) and the social that is of such richness in a clinical archive.

I have indicated several areas to consider in approaching archival research in one's own practice, from the difficult questions of consent and how to maintain confidentiality (particularly for rare cases and places), through addressing the status of the data in the records, to considering a range of potential applications for clinical and sociological purposes. I suggested that the separation of these applications is somewhat artificial as clinical encounters occur between individuals in different positions in a social space, usually of unequal power, holding different perspectives of what should be on research agendas and how these should be tackled. To rely on either an individual practitioner's/researcher's 'integrity' or on a fixed set of guidelines drawn up by any one profession is unlikely to be sufficient or satisfactory: an ongoing and accessible discourse of patients and practitioners is what is needed.

Acknowledgements

Priscilla Alderson has given wise and constructive criticism, advice and encouragement, particularly on the discussion of ethical issues.

Illustrations are reproduced by courtesy of the following, whom I thank: *Figure 4.1* Case History format early 1980s, by kind permission of The British College of Naturopathy and Osteopathy, London; *Figure 4.8* Case History format early 1990s, by kind permission of The British School of Osteopathy, London; *Figure 4.9* Case History format early 1990s, by kind permission of The European School of Osteopathy, Maidstone, Kent; *Figure 4.10* Photograph of Sanne van der Toorn, naturopath and osteopath, at work, 1985, by kind permission of David Hoffman. All other figures were by the author.

Notes

1. The 'strong programme' was outlined by Bloor (1976). The other values the programme is committed to are: (1) *causal* (that is, concerned with the conditions that bring about belief or knowledge states); (2) *impartial* (that is, as sociologists of knowledge we cannot aim to become arbiters of truth or rationality); and (3) *symmetrical* (that is, all knowledge is open to investigation, not just that thought to be 'rejected' or 'irrational').
2. Eric Sotto used this text at a seminar on the relationship between teaching and learning, Open University, Nottingham Regional Centre, 13 September 1995.
3. For example, the notion of 'balanced ligamentous tension' is used to describe the sense of a midpoint of rest (or 'still point') in a patient's limb that one is holding. This can be experienced at any part of the body, for instance just holding an ankle and 'listening' with the hand.

References

Alderson, P. (1992) 'Did Children Change, or the Cuidelines?'. *Bulletin of Medical Ethics* 80: 21–8, August 1992.

Alderson, P. (1995) *Listening to Children: Children, Ethics and Social Research.* Ilford: Barnardo's.

Berthon, J. (1993) 'Research into Archival Data: A Preliminary Report'. *British Osteopathic Journal* 12: 32–9.

Birley, J. (1994) CERES Meeting on Research on Mental Health. Institute of Education, London.

Bloor, D. (1976) *Knowledge and Social Imagery.* London: Routledge and Kegan Paul.

Boruch, R. and Cecil, J. (1979) *Assuring the Confidentiality of Social Research Data.* Philadelphia: University of Pennsylvania Press.

Bourdieu, P. (1990) 'Programme for a Sociology of Sport'. *In Other Words.* Cambridge: Polity Press, pp. 156–7.

Bowling, A. (1991) *Measuring Health.* Milton Keynes: Open University Press.

Britten, N. (1993) 'Record Keeping and Professionalisation in Medicine and Pharmacy'. Paper given at the British Sociological Association Medical Sociology Group conference, York University, September.

Calais-Germain, B. (1993) *Anatomy of Movement.* Seattle, WA: Eastland Press.

Chaplin, E. (1994) *Sociology and Visual Representation.* London: Routledge.

Collins, M. (1994) *A Guide to Audit in Osteopathic Practice.* Reading: The General Council and Register of Osteopaths.

Cooter, R. (1982) 'Anti-contagionism and History's Medical Record', in P. Wright and A. Treacher (eds) *The Problem of Medical Knowledge: Examining the Social Construction of Medicine.* Edinburgh: Edinburgh University Press, pp. 87–108.

Dawes, R. (1988) 'You Can't Systematise Human Judgement: Dyslexia', in J. Dowie and A. Elstein (eds) *Professional Judgement.* Cambridge: Cambridge University Press, pp. 150–62.

Department of Health Circular (1989) HC(89)20.

Einhorn, H. (1988) 'Accepting Error to Make Less Error', in J. Dowie and A. Elstein (eds) *Professional Judgement.* Cambridge: Cambridge University Press, pp. 181–9.

Federation of Feminist Women's Health Centers (1981) *A New View of A Woman's Body.* New York: Simon and Schuster.

Glaser, D. (1985) 'Who Gets Probation and Parole: Case Study versus Actuarial Decision Making'. *Crime and Delinquency* 31: 367–8.

Gombrich, E. H. (1977) *Art and Illusion.* Oxford: Phaidon.

Harrison, B. and Lyon, S. (1993) 'A Note on Ethical Issues in the Use of Autobiography in Sociological Research'. *Sociology* 27(1): 101–9.

Homan, R. (1991) *The Ethics of Social Research.* London: Longman.

Hornibrook, F. A. (1929) *The Culture of the Abdomen.* London: Heinemann.

HMSO (1992) *The Health of the Nation*. London: HMSO.

Jepson, M. (1960) *Anatomical Atlas*. London: John Murray.

Johnson Abercrombie, M. (1989) *The Anatomy of Judgement*. London: Free Association Books, p. 15.

Jupp, V. and Norris, C. (1993) 'Traditions in Documentary Analysis', in M. Hammersley (ed.) *Social Research: Philosophy, politics and practice*. London: Sage, pp. 37–51.

Larner, C. (1984) *Witchcraft and Religion: The Politics of Popular Belief*. Oxford: Blackwell.

Lee, R. (1993) *Doing Research on Sensitive Topics*. London: Sage.

Lockhart, R. (1948) *Living Anatomy*. London: Faber.

Macintyre, S. (1978) 'Some Notes on Record Taking and Making in an Antenatal Clinic'. *Sociological Review* 26(3): 595–611.

McMinn, R. and Hutchings, R. (1988) *A Colour Atlas of Anatomy*. London: Wolfe.

Meehl, P. (1986) 'Causes and Effects of My Disturbing Little Book'. *Journal of Personality Assessment* 50: 370–5.

Melzack, R. and Wall, P. (1982) *The Challenge of Pain*. Harmondsworth: Penguin.

Mendelsohn, K., Nieman, L., Isaacs, K., Lee, S. and Levison, S. (1994) 'Sex and Gender Bias in Anatomy and Physical Diagnosis Text Illustrations'. *Journal of the American Medical Association* 272(16): 1267–70.

Open University (1992) *Professional Judgement and Decision Making*. Milton Keynes: Open University Press.

Pincus, L. and Dare, C. (1980) *Secrets in the Family*. London: Faber.

Place, B. (1993) 'Constructing the Visibility of the Body'. Paper given at the British Sociological Association Medical Sociology Group conference, York University, September.

Power, R. (1991) 'The Whole Idea of Medicine'. PhD thesis, Polytechnic of the South Bank, London.

Power, R. (1994) 'Only nature heals', in S. Budd and U. Sharma (eds) *The Healing Bond*. London: Routledge, pp. 193–213.

Reynolds, P. (1982) *Ethics and Social Research*. New Jersey: Prentice-Hall.

Royal College of Physicians (1990a) *Guidelines on the Practice of Ethics Committees in Medical Research Involving Human Subjects*. London: RCP.

Royal College of Physicians (1990b) *Research Involving Patients*. London: RCP.

Sachs, O. (1987) *The Man Who Mistook His Wife For A Hat*. London: Picador.

Scott, J. (1990) *A Matter of Record*. Cambridge: Polity.

Stacey, M. (1991) 'The Potential of Social Science for Complementary Medicine'. *Complementary Medical Research* 5(3): 183–6.

Stacey, M. (1992) *Regulating British Medicine: the General Medical Council*. Chichester: John Wiley.

Stacey, M. (1994) 'Collective Therapeutic Responsibility: Lessons from the GMC', in S. Budd and U. Sharma (eds) *The Healing Bond*. London: Routledge.

Sykes, J. (ed.) (1982) *The Concise Oxford Dictionary of Current English.* Oxford: Clarendon.

van der Toorn, S. (1983) 'The British College of Naturopathy and Osteopathy Clinic: Facts and Figures: An Analysis of 1,500 Case Histories'. Diploma dissertation. London: BCNO.

Webb, E., Campbell, D., Schwartz, R., Sechrest, L. and Grove, J. (1981) *Non-reactive Measures in the Social Sciences.* Boston: Houghton Mifflin.

Williams, S. (1995) 'Theorising Class, Health and Lifestyles: Can Bourdieu Help Us?'. *Sociology of Health and Illness* 17(5): 577–604.

Wright, P. and Treacher, A. (1982) *The Problem of Medical Knowledge: Examining the Social Construction of Medicine.* Edinburgh: Edinburgh University Press.

Zarzecka, A. and Lorentzon, M. (1995) 'Patients at the London Homoeopathic Hospital 1889–1923'. Paper given at the British Sociological Association Medical Sociology Group conference, York University, September.

Zuckerman, Lord (1961) *A New System of Anatomy.* Oxford: Oxford University Press.

5 Individualized Knowledge: Reflexologists, Biopaths and Kinesiologists in Denmark

Helle Johannessen

Complementary practitioners often claim that each patient must be treated individually. It is presumed that identical symptoms are caused by unique constellations of underlying imbalances in each patient and that the treatment should be tailor-made for the individual. Complementary practitioners usually ascribe a good part of the therapeutic success of their practice to this individualization of treatments. On the other hand, explanations of efficacy in complementary medicine suggested by medical doctors often point to the communication between patient and practitioner as decisive for any therapeutic effect. I would argue that the two positions refer to two facets of the same matter. The clinical conversation is an important tool in the creation of individualized explanations and treatments, and it may be a kind of individualized therapy in itself. In this chapter, I shall present some characteristics of clinical conversations in different clinics and discuss some implications.

Based on participant-observation in clinics of reflexology, biopathy and kinesiology, the making of individualized knowledge is explored. How do practitioners of these three kinds of alternative medicine diagnose? How do they decide what interventions are appropriate for treatment? How is the individualized image, that must precede individualized treatment, created and realized, and what implications does it have in a therapeutic context? For comparison, I include information on procedures for diagnosis and choice of treatment in conventional clinics.

A number of interesting perspectives appear and I have chosen two for further enquiry. First, individuality seems to refer as much to practitioners (complementary and conventional alike) as to patients. Individuality could be considered a general condition of treatment to be recognized and explored in regard to its significance for clinical practice and healing processes. Second, individualized explanations hold great potential for meaning in treatment. When patients get individualized explanations and treatments of the often chronic ailments for which complementary medicine is sought, it is likely to create order in the personal chaos accompanying sickness. This perspective seems interesting because the creation of meaning could be significant not only for the illness experience of the patient but also for healing processes in the patient's body and disease.

Four Scenarios of Diagnosis and Treatment

Let us start by looking at some examples of what happens when patients visit practitioners of various kinds. The central question to be explored is, how is it decided what the problem really is and how it should be dealt with? We start in the well known, in a stereotyped image of a consultation with a medical doctor, and then proceed to equally stereotyped images of consultations with a reflexologist, a biopath and a kinesiologist.[1]

At the Medical Doctor's Office

When a person consults a medical doctor for some health problem the diagnostic process usually proceeds along a general pattern. The patient tells the doctor about symptoms and ailments; the doctor asks more detailed questions regarding these or other possible symptoms that could point to a specific disease. Based on this conversation the doctor develops a hypothesis concerning what disease the patient suffers from and seeks to verify or falsify this hypothesis through physical examinations, laboratory tests and other 'objective' measurements. Eventually a specific diagnosis is decided on and a standard medical treatment is usually prescribed. Of course, other factors are involved in the decision process (for example, the cultural background of the doctor, personal experience, and so on), but let that be for the moment. The point is that a general health examination is not conducted when consulting the doctor for a specific symptom. The conversation and examination is rather selective, conducted in accordance with fundamental principles for diagnosis and treatment taught at medical schools.

In a study of how medical knowledge is structured and passed on to students, Paul Atkinson has shown that medical students are trained to construct a certain type of knowledge in a certain way.

With the patient's report on symptoms as a starting point, the students learn to seek information which can probe that the symptoms refer to a specific disease. Questions and examinations are selected among a multitude of possible questions and examinations on behalf of a hypothesis of what disease could be behind the symptoms (Atkinson 1988). It resembles the work of a detective: the doctor gets a 'clue' (the symptom) and must find the 'offender' (the disease).

It often happens during conversations between medical doctors and patients that information is revealed but not considered important. This counts for patients' verbal communication about worries and other ailments as well as for physical signs noticed by the doctor. Both Atkinson's study and a study of American medical students in a Home Care Program showed that medical students are trained to work along specific patterns of supposed connections between symptoms, diseases and treatment (Atkinson 1988; Sankar 1988). Only the information which is relevant for a presumed disease within this framework is considered. Concerns, relations and physical conditions which may be important for the patient but are not part of the medical framework are left for the patient to deal with on his own.

The medical process of diagnosis and decision on treatment is centred on a disease and restricted to physical symptoms and signs related to this disease within medical science. In the diagnostic process the doctor moves from knowledge of an unspecific condition of an individual patient toward knowledge of a specific condition generalized as a disease. She looks for a predefined formula, a structure, of disease and treatment that suits the patient and can be allotted to him.[2]

At the Reflexologist's Clinic

Consultations with complementary practitioners run along a somewhat different course. The clinical elucidation does not depart from symptoms and is not directed toward definition of a certain disease of the medical system. Quite the contrary, one is tempted to say. Some complementary practitioners prefer not to be informed of symptoms or any medical diagnosis given, so that this knowledge should not interfere with the processes of diagnosis and prescription, the rationale being a belief that causes of seemingly identical symptoms in two or more persons are individual and unique imbalances or functional disturbances of the body system. Within this

rationale, it not possible to deduce anything about the unique con-
stellation of a patient on behalf of symptoms or medically defined
diseases. Instead, the consultation is based on an unravelling of the
general condition of the patient.

When a person consults a reflexologist with a specific problem,
a thorough examination of reflex zones on the feet takes place.[3]
The therapy is based on the assumption that specific zones on the
feet correspond with specific areas of the body at large. On the feet,
a 'map' of the body is recognized, and qualitative differences on
this map are considered signs of differences in functional ability of
body parts. Differences in colours, temperature, dampness, and the
patient's experience of pain, tickling, and so on, in the feet, are
interpreted as signs of the functional ability of corresponding body
parts and form the basis of an individualized explanation and treatment of the problem. Two patients supposedly suffering from the
same disease or medical condition – for example, a headache –
rarely show identical patterns of difference on the feet, partly because the condition of a large number of organs and body systems
is considered.

In reflexology the examination of the reflex zones furthermore
forms the basis of a conversation of daily habits and dispositions.
As the zones are examined corresponding questions are posed by
the reflexologist: for example, regarding eating habits and possible
problems with eating (while massaging zones corresponding with
the stomach), digestion and laxative patterns (at zones of the intes-
tines), amount and kind of beverages taken daily (while working on
the kidney zones), and so on. Even psychological aspects are
touched upon during examination and treatment of the feet. Psychological aspects are usually addressed when zones corresponding
with hormone-producing glands are massaged. If the conversation
reveals inexpedient habits, mental dispositions or physical ailments,
these are all considered elements in the patient's individual health
puzzle and relevant for understanding and treating the present
health problem.

Through the clinical conversation and examination of reflex
zones, the symptoms which brought the patient to the clinic are
woven into a unique and individual pattern including abnormalities
on the reflex zones, functional ability of major organs of the body,
other physical signs and ailments, and daily habits and psycho-
social aspects of the patient. A mental structuration of the patient
and his health problem takes place during this process. The reflexologist does not try to find a predefined formula of disease and
treatment to suit the patient. With the patient she creates a net of

individual dispositions and conditions of the patient that gives conceptual structure and meaning to the situation for both of them. A process of structuration takes place.[4]

Visiting a biopath[5]

Within biopathy an individual diagnosis is obtained by measuring the 'energy' in body meridians and organs as well as the biochemical condition of the patient by the use of an electrical apparatus called a 'biotron'. The biotron is quite similar to the 'Vega tester' used in the German tradition following Dr Voll, but was developed for the use in biopathy by the Danish founder of this medical system. Based originally in Chinese models of correlations between specific acupuncture points, meridians and specific organs of the body, the relative skin resistance in meridian points is interpreted as reflections of the 'energy level' in meridians and organs. By measuring the skin resistance on points of all of twelve main meridians an individual pattern of energy level and functional ability in the major organs of the body is created. The test supposedly reveals individual underlying causes of the symptoms or health problems, and it rarely happens that persons with identical symptoms show identical patterns of energy and functional ability.

This test does not lead directly to treatment but is, anyhow, essential in biopathy. Results of measurements are compared at each consultation by patient and practitioner in collaboration and become tools in the continuous evaluation of the health condition of the patient. From an anthropological perspective, the reading of skin resistance in meridian points puts the body on stage and may in itself be an important therapeutic element. All major body parts are addressed and encompassed in an image of the body and its momentary condition, and the procedure becomes an active part in the process of creating cultural order in the midst of a chaotic sickness episode. A structuration takes place, in the sense that focus points are fixed and structure the patient's experience of body, health condition and therapy.

Biopathic prescriptions consist of diets and herbal and isopathic remedies[6] selected by the use of the biotron. A large number of remedies, food items, allergens (for example, house dust or pollen), and so on, are tested in the biotron to see whether they enhance the functional ability of the body and, therefore, should be included in the prescription. At each consultation more than a hundred remedies are tested, out of which the patient is prescribed between one and twenty. The final combination is rarely identical for two patients even though they may suffer from some identical symptoms.

During biopathic consultations a clinical conversation unfolds along with the reading of the body. The patient is asked about habits and dispositions along with the measuring of energy in meridians and organs, just as during remedy testing. The biopathic conversation does not differ from the reflexological conversation in regard to areas covered. It concerns eating and drinking habits, sleeping habits, laxative patterns, psychological patterns, and so on. Both biopathic and reflexological conversations provide structuration of a multi-levelled and individual pattern of the patient, but the biopathic conversation is more detailed in regard to biochemical aspects.

At the Kinesiologist[7]

In kinesiology the patient's problems and needs of treatment are supposedly revealed through the relative strength of muscles. There are two basic systems of muscle testing. In one system (Touch for Health) the relative strength in 14–48 muscles, supposedly corresponding with specific meridians, organs, biochemical processes and emotions, is tested. It is presupposed that there is correspondence between specific muscles, meridians, organs, biochemical processes and emotions, and during the test an image of energy levels, functional ability in major organs and mental dispositions and conditions is created. In the other basic system (One Brain) the whole test can be performed on one muscle as variations in the relative strength in one muscle are interpreted as digital answers (yes/no, well functioning/malfunctioning, enhances/debilitates, and so on) to questions formulated by the kinesiologist (sometimes not verbally, only mentally). By this procedure kinesiologists believe they can test the body's momentary needs and condition to the extent the bodymind wants to reveal it. It is presupposed that the bodymind knows what and how much it needs now, and that it will answer the kinesiologist's question on behalf of this knowledge.

Prescriptions of treatment are determined by placing remedies on the patient and retesting the strength of formerly 'weak' muscles. If the muscles becomes 'stronger' it is interpreted as a sign that this remedy strengthens the patient. The same procedure can be used for testing food items, conventional medicine, thoughts and emotions. For testing thoughts and emotions the strengths of a muscle are tested while the patient holds certain mental pictures, concentrates on certain emotions or speaks out statements. Variations in strength are interpreted as signs of positive or negative influence of the particular statement, emotions, and so on, on the body system.

The muscle test also functions as an interview guide. When the test reveals low energy or functional ability in a meridian/organ, questions concerning habits and dispositions related to this organ are posed. As psychological and social factors are incorporated in the domain of testing and treating, they are, however, not only topics of conversation but also objects of the clinical test. During kinesiological consultations an individualized image referring to the physical, the biochemical and the mental dimension of the patient's momentary situation and a way out of it is created. Structuration takes place.

Individuality as a Condition

The Patient as a Unique Individual

In the complementary medical systems presented above, an individual multi-levelled health pattern of each patient is created by the means of different techniques for 'reading' the body and the patient. These techniques function both as means for 'objective' registrations of the condition (energy level, functional ability) in each major organ of the body and as interview guides leading patient and practitioner around the subjects of nutrition, digestion, addiction, emotions, and so on. Wide areas of life are touched upon, and it is characteristic that many different factors are designated as co-causes of the actual problem. The findings are rarely presented as a short and precise diagnosis or even summarized at the end of session. Most often, the whole conversation constitutes a complex and individualized diagnosis. Patient and healer select among the many potentials revealed and each chooses that which suits himself and his personal experiences best. A pattern of significance and meaning is created. With the interweaving of many factors into the explanation of the patient's situation, the diagnosis must be individual. One can hardly find two persons with identical constellations of physical, mental and social conditions and dispositions.

The Practitioner as a Unique Individual

Each of the medical systems do, however, also restrict and direct the individualization. Within reflexology the focus is on general physiological characteristics, in biopathy the focus is on biochemical characteristics and in kinesiology much attention is given to mental and psychological characteristics. Furthermore, each practitioner creates a personal variation of the medical systems she practises. This implies that individualization of the patient is only possible within the framework provided by a specific practitioner's personal interpretation and praxis of a specific medical system.

In the clinics I visited, it was obvious that each practitioner worked along personal patterns of diagnosis and prescription. One kinesiologist, for example, diagnosed malfunctioning pancreas in 16 of the 26 patients whose treatment I observed, while this particular problem was not diagnosed in any of 19 patients of another kinesiologist. One biopath revealed masked tuberculosis with 14 of 46 patients, while another biopath only revealed this problem in 1 of 12. Even in something as physical as reflexology, it turned out that practitioners had personal patterns for registering strained reflex zones.

One could be tempted to explain such inter-practitioner variation as conscious manipulation of data by the therapists. But I believe the explanation must be sought in deeply rooted epistemological patterns. Practitioners cannot avoid diagnosing individually, because they themselves are part of the test procedure and their personal preferences and fields of interests are part of the background for the test. Reflexologists feel the feet with their fingers; biopaths control the electrode used for determining skin resistance; the kinesiologist conducts the 'pressing' on the patient's mucles; and all of them interpret the data they produce within their personal theoretical frame of reference. The practitioners do not influence tests and data by purpose but by necessity as they are integral parts of any test performed in the clinic.

My observations of practitioner individuality are supported by controlled trials of complementary test procedures. From persons who have been involved with such trials, I have been told that it has not been possible to reproduce results in two or more independent tests of the same patients. On behalf of these observations, it does not seem viable to maintain the idea that each of the tests are neutral tests of the momentary needs and conditions of the patients. Instead, the test could be conceived as a meeting point between the individual pattern of mental dispositions and techniques of a practitioner and the individual pattern of dispositions in life and body of the patient.

Apart from techniques, each practitioner also has a personal 'style', code of behaviour, charisma, and so on. The range of styles within complementary medicine is as wide as within conventional medicine. One finds any personal blend of the authoritarian, technical, scientific, empathetic, friendly or motherly style. For patients choosing and evaluating practitioners, the style is of utmost importance. It becomes a difference that makes a difference to the choice of practitioner and, according to the patients, also to the therapeutic effect of the treatment.

A general acknowledgement of the individuality of practitioners is reflected in the fact that referrals to complementary practitioners most often are person specific. Complementary practitioners usually try out a number of colleagues by being treated themselves before they select one or two to whom they will refer patients. They wish to know about the others personally and do not consider it enough to know what medical system a person has been trained within. Patients also show great willingness to travel far to consult a practitioner recommended by trustworthy persons. Eventually, patients collect their own experiences of personal techniques and styles of practitioners, and these form the basis of future choices, and it seems that the more experienced patients become within the complementary health care sector, the more consciously they choose not only specific techniques but also specific practitioners.

Individuality and Difference in all Treatment

From a patient perspective the individualization of their health may seem restricted by the framework given through the individuality of practitioners. Some may even feel 'cheated' that the muscle strength, the reflex zones or the biotron do not only provide ultimate (and uninfluenced) messages from one's own bodymind but also reflect the individuality of the practitioner.

From a broader perspective, a very exciting image of individuality – and difference – emerges, a pattern of patients being treated individually (differently) within individual (different) repertoires and styles of practitioners. Individuality seems to refer to patients and practitioners alike and penetrates knowledge and praxis in much complementary medicine. But how about conventional medicine? Is individuality an important quality of that as well?

With regard to individuality and difference of patients, medical science has produced models of, for example, multifactorial relations of cause and effect, biopsychosocial patterns of health, and integration of the patient perspective in clinical work. It does, however, seem that these models have a hard time being implemented in everyday clinical work. The focus is still on identification of standardized and generalized diseases and not on the patient as an individual being in a complex context (Gordon 1988a). Could this be credited to the power of habits (it is hard to change the clinical practice one has been trained and worked in for years)? Or is part of the problem that medical doctors lack concrete tools by which to operationalize the individualistic perspective in a concrete clinical reality? If so, complementary clinical practice could be a rich source of inspiration for development of individualizing clinical procedures.

Though medical science is open to individuality of the patient (at least on a theoretical level), individuality of practitioners seems to conflict with basic medical ideals of praxis. According to the sociological literature on professionalism, homogeneity and standardization of practice are considered central for the medical profession (Freidson 1970). It does, however, seem to be an indisputable fact that conventional medical practice also is subjected to personal and national variations (Gordon 1988b; Payer 1989). Hospitalized patients often recognize that different doctors give different answers, and consciously pose the same question to a number of doctors in their attempt to understand their situation (Jensen et al. 1988). Medical doctors are also individual and different even though they themselves (and the public opinion) usually pretend they are not.

Besides being clinical characteristics, individuality and individualism are central values in Western culture of the present and are important and influential for our actions and ideas. Given high cultural significance, the concepts are laden with potency – they are potentially powerful and working – also in a clinical context. In recognizing this, the individuality of clinical practice need no longer be a taboo. Rather it becomes a culture-bound condition of treatment, and as such should be acknowledged and given attention. We need to explore in depth the significance of individuality for clinical practice and healing processes.

Meaning as Therapy

The multitude of possible explanations and the structuration of unique and individual images of each patient contains an enormous potential for 'meaning' in treatment. Each patient is involved in the structuration of a tailor-made explanation and treatment for whatever problem is brought to the complementary practitioner, which can be very helpful for creating order in the midst of a chaotic illness experience.

People who seek complementary medicine predominantly suffer from pain and allergic symptoms. More than half have been suffering from the same problem for several years (the problems are chronic) and most have been consulting medical doctors or other officially sanctioned practitioners (for example, physiotherapists) without satisfactory effect (Lewith and Aldridge 1991; Brendstrup and Launsþ 1994). There is a continuous chaos in their lives as they must live with their chronic ailments every day for an indefinite period of time, perhaps for ever. For these people, it is often a great relief to visit a complementary practitioner who can reframe their problems and provide for an explanatory model that seems logical and meaningful. Structuration takes place in the patient's mind as order and meaning are created.

Among the 286 'complementary' patients interviewed in this study, more than 65 per cent reported on effect of the therapy, and interestingly there is no significant variation in 'effect score' for the individual practitioners. How could it be possible? What could explain that patients are relieved from relatively similar symptoms (pain in the musculo-skeletal system, headaches, eczema, asthma, fatigue) by treatments based on an individual diagnosis framed within the highly individualized knowledge and skills of a (random) practitioner?

Could it be that the central issue is not what therapy and explanation is provided, but rather that explanation and therapy is provided? Could the issue of meaning be of therapeutic significance in regard to both the illness experience of the patient and the pathological disease? This is a new perspective, which demands systematic investigation before potential relations can be more clearly defined. But it is a promising perspective, in the sense that it holds potential for a scholarly explanation of much of that which is presently dumped into the black-box of placebo. Let me briefly sketch some outlines for this.

Placebo and Meaning

In a study of research on the effect of complementary medicine, especially spiritual/psychic healing, the Dutch researcher Sybo Schouten concluded that both placebo and much complementary medicine seem to have more effect on patients' general feeling of well-being than on specific diseases. In support of this, he argued that there is no significant difference in the effectiveness of various complementary modes of healing in regard to non-life-threatening diseases; that both complementary medicine and placebo can give objectively measurable effects to a lesser extent, possibly as a consequence of improved well-being and thereby increased self-regulating capacity in the body; that subjective improvements seem to be more pronounced than objectively measurable improvements in complementary medicine as well as in placebo; and that psychological variables, especially associated with the patient and with the patient–healer relationship, seem to be correlating with effects (Schouten 1992–93).

Psychological variables associated with the patient and with the patient–healer relationship are often interpreted as the patient's 'blind faith' in complementary treatment, and as practitioners paying lip-service to the patient's point of view. These interpretations do not, however, correspond with the material I collected among Danish patients and practitioners. It would be a gross simplification to state that the practitioners only tell patients what they want to hear. The explanations offered are most often logical and probable to the patient as they draw upon general cultural models, but the practitioners deliver something other than what is expected by patients. Many patients explain that they have gained insight into new areas of health and healing and, thus, have gained a new perspective on their own health through consultations with complementary medicine. To explain the effects of complementary medicine by referring to the 'blind faith' of patients seems similarly irrelevant since it is characteristic of complementary patients that they have greater faith in medical doctors and their therapeutic skills than in complementary practitioners and their skills. Many have already tried various options within the conventional medical systems without satisfactory help, but this does not lead them to believe firmly in miraculous healing in complementary medicine. Rather, patients are pragmatic; they are willing to 'give it a try' with some complementary mode of treatment since the conventional therapies do not seem to work for them.

The psychological variables more likely refer to a conscious co-acting of patients and practitioners. The treatment works best if the patient is co-realizing, co-knowing, co-deciding and co-creating in the process of diagnosis and treatment. A new picture is structured by patient and practitioner in collaboration; an individual and meaningful image which to many becomes more important than getting rid of the symptoms. One patient who sought reflexology because of pain thus told me: 'It [reflexology] helped a lot. Not so much on the pain, but on my mental balance. For a long time I was able to handle everything in a different way, and that made me believe in it [the treatment form].'

This example illustrates that we may even be dealing with an anti-expectation effect, or a 'turning everything upside-down and looking at from a new perspective' effect. A new and unexpected order is created in the chaos of sickness.

The validity of the Danish material is supported by findings of the American anthropologist/sociologist Meredith McGuire in a study of alternative healing in the suburbs of New Jersey. McGuire concluded that the main common characteristic of patients who have been helped by alternative or complementary medicine was that some kind of order was created in their personal lives. For these persons symptoms and other aspects of life were connected in a narrative that gave meaning to it all. Analogous with this, McGuire stated that changes in identity and self are more important than physical improvements when patients evaluate the 'success' of a treatment (McGuire 1995).

Meaning, Illness and Disease

Changes in the patient's perception of his health problems, himself and his situation in general refers to the illness perspective in the distinction between illness and disease which has been prevalent in medical anthropology for the past few years (see, for example, Kleinman 1980). The illness, the patient's psycho-social experience of the sickness episode, becomes less chaotic when a symbolic order is created, and symbolic order is exactly what is created during body readings and clinical conversations in complementary medicine. The process of symbolic structuration continues beyond the initial consultation – through repeated consultations and in the patient's mind between consultations. For patients the issues raised with the complementary practitioner echo into everyday life with habits and dispositions unfolding in praxis, being suppressed, resisted, enhanced, and so on, on behalf of the health pattern created at the complementary clinic. Pain is no longer something to avoid by all means, but becomes a sign in the body language. It is given meaning and 'tells' the patient something about his life at this very moment. To drink water is no longer just a thirst-reducing action; it becomes a tool for cleansing the body. It is given meaning and becomes a part of therapy. Changes in the illness perspective point to changes in the quality of life. The more meaning that can be attributed to the sickness episode and everyday life, the higher the potential for quality of life, in the sense that anxiety and confusion are lessened and potentials of relevant actions are enhanced. But what about the disease perspective? Could meaning also influence that?

As already mentioned, most analyses of complementary medicine suggest that subjectively experienced improvements are more pronounced than objectively measurable ones. This implies, however, that there is some objective effect: in some instances, without significance relative to a placebo-treated control group; in others, significantly more effect than in control groups. Part of the effect can possibly be explained by specific effects of the therapies (the massage on the reflex zone or the chemical substances in a herbal remedy) – these issues are being researched by a growing number of scientists around the world. But in many instances it proves difficult to define specific relations of cause and effect, and it seems plausible to speak of the effect as being primarily caused by non-specific or indirect factors. Meaning-producing structuration could be one of these.

This rather bold suggestion is probed by research in psycho-neuro-immunology (PNI) and self-healing processes in the body. Within PNI it has convincingly been demonstrated that psychological processes, the central nervous system and the immune system are linked and influence each other. Based on PNI research we can state that

> there is little doubt, that emotional strain and stressful stimuli are able to influence the immune response with possible health consequences; and ... it is probable that psychological stimulation in the form of hypnosis, relaxation and guided imagery techniques may influence the immune response significantly .... (Zacharia 1994: 236)

A problem with research within PNI is that it is laboratory based and experimental. The influence of specific mental techniques on specific bodily activities is being researched, but we lack research and knowledge of the relation between mental processes in life and biological processes in the body. The lessening of anxiety and confusion and the enhanced potential for action as supported by meaning-producing structuration (in life) could perhaps be parallel to the relaxation and mental focusing induced by specific mental techniques (in PNI research). I suggest meaning and structuration as general mental aspects that can possibly influence biological processes through the complex communication systems of the body.

A quite different issue which is central to this discussion is whether objective registrations are more important for health than subjective experiences. I believe it can be assumed not to be so. By now, many studies have shown that in a population with identical symptoms only half (or even less) seek medical advice or help. Objective symptoms, disease and treatment are not correlating parameters and cannot be directly deduced from each other. To some persons, life apparently is orderly enough not to seek medical help (they have no illness), though a pathological chaos (a disease) can be detected. Furthermore, many complementary patients do not show any pathological chaos. In much chronic pain and the 'diffuse symptoms' from which many complementary patients suffer, there is no 'disease' to cure, no 'objective parameters' to monitor. The chaos is, therefore, not primarily pathological but psycho-social, which points further to the relevance of meaning-producing structuration as therapy in itself. Meaning can create order in a psycho-social chaos, and individualized knowledge can produce meaning.

Notes

1. Where no reference is given, the data have been produced during my fieldwork in the alternative sector of the Danish health care system, 1989–91. Data were collected by participant observation and ethnographic interview. The project was financed by the Danish Research Councils of the Humanities, Medicine and Social Sciences and was carried out at the Institute of Anthropology, University of Copenhagen. A full report of the study is published in Johannessen (1994).
2. In this text I use 'she' for practitioners to remind people that many practitioners are women, though we often think of experts as males, and 'he' for patients to remind people that many patients are men, though the majority in fact are women.
3. Reflexology can be centred on reflex zones situated in different body parts: the feet, the hands, the nose, the back, and so on. In Denmark, foot reflexology is by far the most common form of reflexology, and in this chapter I deal only with this kind of reflexology as it is being practised in Denmark.
4. Editor's note: the term 'structuration' is used here to refer to a different process from that to which the sociologist Anthony Giddens has applied the term.
5. Biopathy is a special kind of naturopathy that has evolved in Denmark since the early 1980s. The therapy combines German traditions of electro-acupuncture, diluted medical remedies and dietism with American traditions of vitamin- and mineral-therapy as well as older Scandi-

navian traditions of herbal medicine. Biopathy is probably the medical system with focus on natural remedies and diluted medications that is presently most common in Denmark.

6. Isopathic remedies are potentized medical substances, similar to homoeopathic remedies, but while homoeopathic remedies relate to whole constellations of symptoms and dispositions, isopathic remedies relate to single symptoms, organs or disease agents.

7. In many countries kinesiology seems to be a technique included in the clinical repertoire by a number of different kinds of practitioners, perhaps especially chiropractors. In Denmark kinesiology has, on the contrary, developed into a medical system of its own, with schools, professional associations, and so on, and the title of kinesiologist refers to practitioners basing their clinical practice primarily on the muscle test.

References

Atkinson, Paul (1988) 'Discourse, Descriptions and Diagnoses: Reproducing Normal Medicine', in M. Lock and D. Gordon (eds) *Biomedicine Examined*. Dordrecht/Boston/London: Kluwer Academic Press, pp. 179–204.

Brendstrup, E. and Launsþ, L. (1994) *Research on Alternative Medicine in Denmark. A Literature Study* [in Danish]. Copenhagen: National Board of Health.

Freidson, E. (1970) *The Profession of Medicine. A Study in the Sociology of Applied Knowledge*. New York: Dodd, Mead and Co.

Gordon, D. (1988a) 'Tenacious Assumptions in Western Medicine', in M. Lock and D. Gordon (eds) *Biomedicine Examined*. Dordrecht/Boston/London: Klewer Academic Press, pp. 19–56.

Gordon, D. (1988b) 'Clinical Science and Clinical Expertise: Changing Boundaries Between Art and Science in Medicine', in M. Lock and D. Gordon (eds) *Biomedicine Examined*. Dordrecht/Boston/London: Kluwer Academic Press, pp. 257–95.

Jensen, S. S., Neilsen, H., Samuelson, H. and Steffen, V. (1988) *What is the Meaning of Cancer? A Study Among Danish Patients and Practitioners* [in Danish]. Copenhagen: The Danish Cancer Society.

Johannessen, H. (1994) *Complex Bodies. Alternative Medicine in Anthropological Perspective* [in Danish]. Copenhagen: Academic Press.

Kleinman, A. (1980) *Patients and Healers in the Context of Culture*. Berkeley: University of California Press.

Lewith, G. and Aldridge, D. (eds) (1991) *Complementary Medicine and the European Community*. Saffron Walden: The C.W. Daniel Co. Ltd.

McGuire, M. (1995) 'Alternative Therapies: The Meaning of Bodies in Knowledge and Practice' in H. Johannessen, J. Andersen and S. Olesen (eds) *Studies in Alternative Therapy 2. Body and Nature*. Odense: Odense University Press, pp. 15–32.

Payer, L. (1989) *Medicine and Culture. Notions of Health and Sickness in Britain, the US, France and West Germany*. London: Victor Gollancz.

Sankar, A. (1988) 'Patients, Physicians and Context: Medical Care in the Home', in M. Lock and D. Gordon (eds) *Biomedicine Examined*, Dordrecht/Boston/London: Kluwer Academic Press, pp. 155–78.

Schouten, S. (1992–93) 'Psychic Healing and Complementary Medicine'. *European Journal of Parapsychology* 9: 35–91.

Zacharia, B. (1994) 'Mind, Immunity and Psychological Intervention: Experimental Studies and Clinical Perspectives', in H. Johannessen, *et al.* (eds) *Studies in Alternative Therapy 1. Contributions from the Nordic Countries*. Odense: Odense University Press, pp. 227–39.

PART THREE

Individual Bodies and the Body Politic: Issues of Empowerment

Many complementary medical practitioners tend to emphasize the equal and non-hierarchical relationship between the patient and practitioner and some therapists hold it as a matter of conviction that patients ought to be actively involved in their treatment, so that the encounter becomes a learning as well as a healing process. This view of the therapeutic-encounter description can be contrasted with orthodox medical encounters where it is often suggested that the patient's perspective is not given such serious attention. Commentators have argued that orthodox medicine is mechanistic, seeing the patient purely as a 'case' of some disease or disorder. The absence of the idea that the patients are active sense-making individuals, who have a contribution to make to their own healing experience, means that effectively the patient may be reduced to a position of deference and dependency. Social scientists have also pointed to the ever expanding medicalization of our social lives and the role of the medical profession to survey and control the public. These ideal types suggest that orthodox and complementary medicine operate at different ends of an empowerment spectrum.

Helen Busby's chapter certainly supports such a portrayal. Chinese Chi Kung is a self-healing practice now taught in parts of Britain and gives to the patient an alternative framework for knowing their body. Busby shows how the expert and the lay individual are equally involved in the healing process and the exchange of information. A kind of empowerment is effected by offering individuals resources for the interpretation of their experiences which do not by-pass subjectivity.

Nevertheless, it is also possible to suggest that complementary medical knowledge supports a surveillance function. Espen Braathen offers such a reading of the role of complementary medical knowledge in his discussion of homoeopathy. Offering patients more responsibility for their own healing may represent empowerment at the level of the individual but at the collective level may be seen as a means by which populations are enlisted in a process of 'self-disciplining'.

These two chapters suggest that the role of complementary medical knowledge is no less contradictory than that of the orthodox clinic.

6 Alternative Medicines / Alternative Knowledges: Putting Flesh on the Bones (Using Traditonal Chinese Approaches to Healing)

Helen Busby

This chapter explores the experience and knowledge of a group of predominantly white English people learning a Chinese self-healing practice known as Chi Kung. In it I attempt to merge pragmatic with cultural questions, to see (potential) users of alternative therapies as people who may make cultural meanings as well as seeking help. In doing so, I am inspired by the paradigm of embodiment, so eloquently proposed by Csordas, as a methodological framework. Associated with this framework is

> the methodological postulate that the body is not an object to be studied in relation to culture, but is to be considered as the subject of culture, or in other words, as the existential ground of culture. (Csordas 1990: 5)

The embodiment paradigm, then, involves an attempt to develop an anthropology 'not only of the body but from the body' (Csordas 1994: xi). Taking the fact of our experiencing life in and through our bodies, it is argued, enables us fruitfully to reconsider aspects of social life including, for example, experiences of disablement or of chronic pain. It is argued that the potential of the embodiment paradigm is wider in scope than traditionally 'medical' topics; that classic themes of concern to social theorists can be reconsidered. Part of this potential lies in the possibility of using life as experienced through the body as the basis for reconsidering such entrenched dualities as those of body/mind, and subject/object. Whilst it is not possible to put forward the approach in depth here, it is intended that this chapter will 'embody' the approach, and illustrate its potential as a focus for developing an analysis of social phenomena.

I extend the concept of medical pluralism, initially coined by anthropologists to suggest the use of a whole range of therapeutic options by people seeking help in 'developing' countries, to include the idea of a plurality of knowledges from which the contemporary Western European consumer[1] may draw. I draw on interviews and dialogues with the group of Chi Kung students/practitioners, all of whom also had some other experience of non-orthodox approaches to healing.

The wide range of groups undertaking healing in the UK during the two or three hundred years preceding the 1858 Medical Registration Act is well documented (see, for example, Saks, this volume). We cannot know (though we could speculate) the extent to which people continued to use non-biomedical healing practices between that point and the more recent past. However, there is now a consensus that consumer interest in and use of alternative medicines is numerically significant and is increasing. This gives rise to an important question about the nature of the relationship between consumers or potential consumers and their 'alternative' practitioners.[2] This little addressed question forms the backdrop to my research.

In attempting to consider the social significance of alternative medicines and methods of healing in contemporary European societies, we face an inherent dilemma: there is a risk, even a likelihood, of blurring together a whole range of phenomena which have little in common other than their exclusion at this point in time from mainstream medicine. There is an argument that the significance of each therapy should be considered and researched in its own right, separately perhaps. On the other hand, the growing interest in and increasingly high profile of alternative forms of healing generally has been plausibly related to wider social movements or shifts (see, for example, Pietroni 1990; Benoist and Cathebras 1993; Douglas 1994). In order to keep in mind these broader issues, I have also used the Chi Kung group as a locus for a more general exploration of the use of a range of healing practices (by the same group). The range of activities from undertaking particular bodily practices to the seeking of help from alternative practitioners is viewed as a continuum, with the former potentially informing the latter, and the relationship with the practitioner is seen as being dynamic because the consumer will always bring some knowledge and meaning to bear on it.

The Research Setting

This consideration of how people engage with the knowledges implicit in alternative medicines is grounded in a small local study. This chapter represents only an initial exploration of these issues, which are being further developed elsewhere.

The study itself was conducted with a group of people in Brighton attending a summer school in the summer of 1993 at Brighton Natural Health Centre (BNHC). BNHC is an educational charity providing classes in a wide range of movement-based and other holistic approaches for people in the community. Brighton itself is known for its cultural diversity, and its plethora of alternatives in medicine and healing. In common with many towns in the UK, a range of healing traditions, both indigenous and brought by travellers and immigrants, have been available and influential at different times. Currently, hundreds, perhaps thousands of practitioners of homoeopathy, acupuncture, herbal medicine, reflexology, aromatherapy, rebirthing, and many others, jostle for customers.

Because the principles underlying Chi Kung are in such sharp contrast to those underlying biomedicine, the question of how people who are interested in such a practice deal with the tension between the one system and another – if they do – comes into sharper focus. In addition, their undertaking of a bodily practice would, I thought, make it more possible for me to ask questions about how they experienced and thought about their bodies. This was not a study 'about' Chi Kung, but one which used the context of a Chi Kung class as a microcosm, to draw on the experiences of people who I (correctly) expected would have been exposed to a variety of ways of thinking about and working with the body.

Stance

The ethos of the research was ethnographic. (Ethnographic research is characterized by the first-hand study of a small community. Observational methods, including participant observation, are used, with the aim of developing a 'thick description' (Geertz 1973) of a particular society – or part of a society – in other words, a multilayered description of social life.) In accordance with the openness of this stance, my aim was to explore the experiences of a small group of people who had some involvement with alternative forms of healing. The issue of interweaving different forms of knowledge about the body emerged from their contributions in the interviews as a crucial, vibrant issue.

By participating in the group myself, I was able to experience some of the struggles (physical and conceptual) which my interviewees talked about. Recently, an awareness of the anthropologist/researcher as embodied has been made more explicit (see, for example, Okely 1993). This is nowhere more pertinent than in the case of anthropologists working in a medical or health context, where social scientists may be so 'at home' with many of the 'tenacious assumptions' (Gordon 1988) of Western biomedicine that they may taken them for granted, or embody them, rather than consciously considering or analysing them.

In addition to participating in Chi Kung classes over approximately four months, and having informal discussions with participants, I conducted twelve in-depth (tape recorded) interviews, each lasting between one and a half and two hours. Equal numbers of men and women were interviewed, their ages ranging from late teens to late fifties. All were white British, except for one young black man whose parents were of Afro-Caribbean origin. Apart from one former antiques dealer who was unemployed, their occupations included teaching, self-employment and being a full-time student. As a group, they ascribed considerable importance to having control over the nature of their work and working environment, even where this meant having a lower income. (Many were on a low income even whilst working, and would be difficult to classify using conventional categories of social class.) Where I have used quotations from the interviews in the text below, I have selected them for the way in which they illustrate or encapsulate themes which were recurrent. In other words, I have drawn from what is common ground amongst the participants in the group, rather than from the many ways in which they are different.

The interviews began by my asking about the class which the person was attending, which in most cases was the Chi Kung class: I asked how they felt when they were doing the Chi Kung, how they came to be doing it, and I used this as a starting point for exploring how they experienced their bodies. These questions often provided enough material for someone to talk for an hour, in terms of a narrative about health. I also asked what they did to stay well or, when they were unwell, what kinds of healing practices they (had) used, whether they had enough energy for their activities (or some other question leading into discussing 'energy'), what they thought about the idea of 'Chi' in Chinese medicine (all were familiar with this term) and whether there were any tensions between the ideas they now had about health and the ones that they had grown up with.

In a wider sense, the participant observation could be said to have begun prior to the study itself, as I had been immersed in the cultural life of Brighton and its alternative healers for many years.

Chi Kung

Chi Kung, together with acupuncture and herbal medicine, forms a part of the traditional systems of healing in China. Having gained in popularity in China in recent years (Ots 1994), it is currently taught in medical contexts to people with serious disease, and also undertaken by many people who practise in order to maintain health. Within the past ten to fifteen years, some of the techniques and practices of Chi Kung have been brought to Europe by practitioners or teachers who have emigrated, and by interested visitors returning from China. Rather than making any attempt to describe the history of Chi Kung, I will outline several features of the practice which were held to be significant by my interviewees and different from many exercise classes which they had attended (but similar in some respects to classes in Tai Chi and Yoga).

What struck me each time I watched a group of people practising Chi Kung was a rare sense of stillness.[3] Each movement is performed with great deliberation, slowly. Students are instructed to harmonize movements with their own breathing, and to cultivate an awareness of their breathing and their bodies. Each new movement is taught with an image: for example, in one movement involving the gradual raising of arms, class members were asked to imagine a wave coming up behind them, so that their arms were carried up effortlessly by the wave (or by the use of the image to direct the Chi). Images are vital to the teaching and philosophy of Chi Kung, rooted as it is in Taoist philosophies, with their central tenet of observing and learning from nature, and the central image of the water flowing towards its inevitable destination, the sea, but adapting to the terrain, whether it be boulders, mountain or other obstacles.

When I asked my interviewees to describe how they felt during any single movement, they usually described the standing pose, which they were asked to adopt for up to fifteen minutes at a time. There are particular details in the instructions about the stance, such as the slight bending of the knees, which demand a continuous effort. Yet most people described the standing as intensely peaceful.

'A Healing Journey'

The metaphor of a healing journey was used by many of the participants as they described a change from relying on conventional medical knowledge and practice to using and drawing upon a range of alternative practices. Some had suffered from severe illness or disease in the conventional sense; others had been impelled not by physical illness, but by a sense of alienation, to seek wholeness through healing practices. Two viewed their practice as being motivated by the need to relax at work, but only one was a resolute pragmatist with no interest in the wider aspects of the practice. Most saw biomedicine primarily as a welcome resource for emergencies where the body was profoundly damaged through injury or accident, or where surgery could resolve what was seen to be the cause of the illness. All had at some point consulted an alternative practitioner; some had consulted a wide range of practitioners.

The following individual 'case study' illustrates some of the complexities of the learning by a person of white English ethnicity[4] of a Chinese self-healing practice. On the one hand, there is a perception of the 'foreignness' of a practice like Chi Kung, with all its strange words and ideas about the body; on the other hand, there is a sense of alienation, not only from Western biomedical practice but also to some extent from its reductionism, and a sense of 'coming home' to a practice which is in some ways more congruent with one's experience of the body.

Synthesizing Meaning: Teresa

'I've sort of been thinking that in Chinese medicine and philosophy you've got these lines in the body which we in the Western world have really not ... and I'm really struck with the acupuncture as to how its helped with the back pain, and how they can use acupuncture as an anaesthetic like a normal operation ...

So to my mind there are definitely things that Western medicine doesn't explain, and so, when talking about energy, my initial feeling is er, well, that all seems very odd, you know, that's my arm which has got some veins going through it and sort of flesh and bones. Why should there particularly be energy channels? But on the other hand, I can't explain the acupuncture, and so I'm quite prepared to accept that there are energy flows in the body. ...' (Teresa)

Teresa's words above indicate a process of struggling to understand and integrate unfamiliar concepts about 'energy'. Teresa's situation was particularly pertinent because she had only very recently come into contact with these ideas about her body, which form part of Traditional Chinese Medicine (TCM), and also perhaps because the acuteness of her situation gave her account, to me, a particular sense of immediacy and change.

Four weeks before I interviewed her, Teresa had attended her first acupuncture treatment, and her presence at the Chi Kung class resulted from her practitioner's recommendation that she attend it. She had sought acupuncture treatment at her physician's recommendation, to help with back pain which was thought to be associated with secondary cancer in her liver.

During our interview she described to me how, three years previously, she had undergone surgery for the treatment of recently diagnosed bowel cancer, and felt confident that 'the cancer had just been cut away and that was it'. Several years later, Teresa was given a course of chemotherapy for secondary cancer, and said that she was then told that Western medicine had little else to offer, although she should come back when she felt worse. Her account of her initial treatments was one of surprising discoveries. In her description of her treatment, she emphasized that whereas she expected to have needles inserted in her back, around the areas where she had experienced pain, she also had needles inserted on her calves and feet, areas considered unrelated to back pain in Western anatomy and physiology. When she asked her acupuncturist why he did this, he explained that these were points on a liver meridian. In her observation of the location of particular points, and her acupuncturist's explanation of these, came Teresa's introduction to a previously unknown system of physiology.

She described how her acupuncturist had explained to her that, in order to have some benefit:

'the needles need to go down until you have some sort of sensation; it's not exactly painful, but as he puts the needles in, there suddenly comes a point where you're conscious, it feels as though you're hitting something, and at that point I say yes ... and all the needles are adjusted to that point'. (Teresa)

The feeling as the needles go in is (interpreted as) the Chi responding; this response is considered essential to the treatment process. In TCM, disharmonies of Chi are considered responsible for illness and disease. In China, this is widely learnt as part of everyday knowledge about the body; in England, and other European societies where acupuncture is practised, it is a concept with which many people are unfamiliar, and is more often learnt through the treatment process itself.

Teresa also emphasized the pleasurable aspects of the treatment: for example, the experience of having moxibustion (which involves burning herbs on the skin at particular points) 'which sounded alarming' but was 'just a very nice soothing session, and the nice smell of the herbs'.

Feeling very weak after her chemotherapy, Teresa had felt that she needed a 'tonic' of some kind and had attempted to discuss this with her consultant, with little success. When her acupuncturist explained that the herbs used in TCM to treat cancer were a combination of herbs which were 'toxic' (to the cancer) and others which are intended to be tonic, she was very relieved to find that Chinese medicine had a way of understanding and working with this need which she felt. In this, and in other ways, there was a sense in which the Chinese approach, although not a part of her indigenous culture, was more congruent with her experience of the body than the biomedical approach.

Alternative Medicines: Alternative Knowledges?

I owe the origins of this chapter in part to an anthropologist who asserted to me that the vast majority of English people having acupuncture treatment would do so for pain relief or alleviation of other symptoms, without engaging with the 'bizarre' and unfamiliar concepts about the body underlying the practice, which could have little relevance to them. Yet Teresa's account illustrates that such an engagement with a different paradigm may be more common than this view asserts. I knew that I myself, having sought treatment from a cranial osteopath and subsequently from an acupuncturist as a result of experiencing a sense of ('physical') pain which biomedicine seemed to have no knowledge to reach, had experienced both practitioners as helping me to piece my scattered body together, with their knowledge about how experiences of the body related to each other being essential to this process. A brief account of this experience is included here in the spirit of going beyond 'participant observation' towards a stance of 'experiencing participation' (Ots 1994: 134), a shift which has been called for by a number of anthropologists working within the embodiment paradigm.

In the case of the cranial osteopath, whom I had consulted for chronic and severe head pain, the problem was diagnosed as being at the level of fluid circulating in the spinal column, which was said to be blocked in a particular way. The acupuncturist, whom I consulted for a sense of deep and overwhelming exhaustion, responded with a strategy of nourishing Blood and Chi. In both cases, the explanations seemed to fit with my experience, and it would be difficult for me to separate the conceptual from the physical interventions (that is, the gentle manipulation of my neck in the first case and the insertion of needles in the second). The experience of pain as being inchoate and alienating from one's own body, and the importance of developing an explanation/narrative as an element of surviving/healing has been explored in a number of phenomenological accounts (for example, Sacks 1984; Kleinman et al. 1992). In the embodiment paradigm, knowledge is seen as being synthesized within the body, rather than being an external or mental explanatory framework. Embodied 'synthesis of meaning' (Csordas 1990) will take place within the context of a range of practices, including biomedicine and a number of alternative therapies.

Both the practices I have referred to work with concepts of the body which fly in the face of medical science. Cranial osteopaths aim to work on the movements of the joints between the cranial bones, and on the circulation of the cerebrospinal fluid, using a radical reinterpretation of orthodox anatomy. The rich and complex ideas underlying acupuncture and TCM are documented elsewhere (Kaptchuk 1983), and although neurophysiological explanations for some aspects of the treatment have been proposed, they arguably overlook the complexity of the practice (Saks 1992). The idea, based in TCM, of nourishing of Blood and Chi energy which appealed to me seems to link into a wider 'lay' concern with energy in my own (British) culture.

Having been involved in the culture of Brighton's alternative healers, it seemed to me that many therapies invited a reshaping of one's way of thinking about the body, and that this issue was a wider one than the specific cultural differences between 'East' and 'West' implicit in the use by white European patients of traditional Chinese medicine. Power's (1994) description of some of the key features of naturopathy, with its underlying tenet of 'letting nature heal' reveals another example of this. An implication of this philosophy for many naturopathic practitioners is a commitment not to prescribe remedies or medicines, an injunction she describes as sometimes truly challenging to practitioner and patient alike. In my reading of her work, it is not only the non-prescribing which is challenging, but also the grasping of the idea of an intelligent 'nature' within the body, so contradictory to the mechanistic version of biomedical physiology and pathology.

'Energy'

The focus of much of the informal conversation between classes at BNHC was a discussion about bodily experiences, and there was an emphasis on the importance of the inner body. Teresa said that she had undergone a change from assessing her body primarily in terms of performance to thinking about it in terms of how it feels. Others commented on a similar transition; one man commented that he used to exercise to 'look good', whereas now he exercised more for a sense of balance.

The concept of energy was used to explore the possibility of a dynamic life-force which underlies all bodily manifestations, including sensations, disorders/diseases, and other experiences in the body, such as a sense of connectedness. Mathew said he felt dizzy every time he began the Tai Chi, but less so each day. On the first day he could hardly stand, he said, but he could stand more easily by the second class. On this day, he experienced hot and cold flushes all over his body. On other days he experienced sweating in different parts of his body, and on the day I interviewed him he had felt a tingling sensation all over his body during the class. After the classes, he felt as though he had been 'flushed out', he felt 'clearer', and more able to carry on with his day.

Similar accounts of experiences of heat and tingling are often found in the literature about healing practices; Csordas (1993), in his work on American Catholic charismatic healers, refers to such experiences. In this context, he emphasizes the importance of not bypassing the bodily synthesis of meaning by imposing, for example, the physiological concept of sensation as a core explanation. In my example, it would not be difficult to find physiological explanations for participants' experiences. Mathew had been diagnosed at birth as suffering from a serious heart condition which had necessitated repeated surgery throughout his life, and which he associated with a pervasive feeling of weakness. In the context of practising Chi Kung, however, he experienced the weakness, tingling, and so on, as part of a therapeutic process, rather than simply as a symptom.

The people I interviewed chose to view their experiences more as a manifestation of energy which was associated with a life-force of some kind. Although this concept of a life-force is poorly developed in British society, it was, for this group, a real if elusive concept. Anthony explained it thus:

'The way I experienced it – if you put your arms in the Chi Kung position – I could feel a sort of magnetic, elastic feeling between my arms, but also some sort of flow.
I think a lot of people read God into it or something like that ... but I actually think it's more like there is just a flow going around, and it's more natural – my body's another instrument or tool, and it's not always tuned in, but when it is, it perceives that flow more.' (Anthony)

Not all the participants were as comfortable with the idea of energy:

'I have a really big struggle with things like "energy flows", you know, lines going through ....' (Angie)

Angie was referring to the belief that Chi animates and flows through the body. She was not alone in finding this and its corollary concepts puzzling and problematic. My interviews with people attending the class enabled me to enquire about their views at the point where they were struggling to relate them to/reconcile them with other views about the body and about healing. Although in this case, the terminology of a non-indigenous form of healing highlights the conceptual struggle, being confronted with the idea of energy or life-force is an experience which may occur in many cases of consultation with alternative practitioners.

Chi Kung and the Western Habitus

Whilst some healing practices may transform the phenomenological world of the practitioner/patient, others may rather be said to dissolve some of its features or foundations. Bourdieu (1977) used the term 'habitus' to denote the way in which the body stores and reproduces patterns and potentials which are culturally specific. Self-control, discipline, alienation and fragmentation have all been suggested as key themes characterizing the 'Western'[5] habitus, by Crawford (1985), Marx – interpreted by Scarry (1985) – and Martin (1987), respectively. Whilst not uncontested, the metaphor of the body as machine is a dominant one in the industrialized countries of Western Europe and the US.

Participants in the classes at BNHC experienced their process of learning as simultaneously being one of unlearning. Sophie said that she felt the awareness of her body that she was beginning to find was 'something which should be natural' but was 'blocked' by the 'kind of work ethic' she had grown up with, which meant that she must always be active. Perhaps the most specific unlearning entailed by those learning practices like Chi Kung is the instruction to be aware of the 'inner body' during practice. (The ability on the part of Chinese people to report minute details about changes within their bodies is commonly reported by Western observers and researchers in China (Farquhar 1991). The Chinese habitus, we may conclude, comprises a different range of norms about awareness of the body than the 'Western' habitus. Western Europeans may be able to report on changes in their bodies in such detail, but they would probably be referred to as being 'hypochondriac' or 'somatizing'.)

The difference between the Chi Kung class and some other kinds of exercise classes was noted by almost everyone I talked to.

'it seems to me that, you know, dance classes are very disciplined, and quite – not violent, that's not the right word, but something like that'.

'this is a more kind of natural way ... it's a more kind of balanced exercise; it's not going to one extreme and then relaxing, it's more of a flow'.

When new movements were introduced by the teacher, they were associated with images or concepts. Each sequence was broken down into very simple movements, each to be carried out with either an inhalation or while breathing out. The length of time taken to do the movement should correspond to the breath, so that the time taken will vary from one person to another; it is this rhythm of one's own breathing which ideally shapes one's progress through the movements, and not the urge to keep up with the person in front.

Implicit in the teaching of Chi Kung which I observed is a paradox: the emphasis is on allowing a relaxed openness, for the Chi to circulate, and yet the requirements of (regular) practise and the details of the movements require considerable discipline. Very detailed instructions are given about how to stand and, although the standing position could become uncomfortable if held for longer than a short time, the teacher advised staying in the position for some time, and only stopping if compelled to. Amongst the members of the group, there was a considerable emphasis on disciplines, routines and regimens of caring for the body and the self, some of which were taken for granted. It was my impression that there was a discourse about caring for oneself which merged some distinctively modern European elements (the emphasis on discipline) with some traditional Chinese images and ideals (the life-source flowing, like a river, to its ultimate destination). In the eyes of those I interviewed, this discipline was a gentle one, used not to enhance productivity, but to pursue their own ends, which were defined variously as spiritual enlightenment, pleasure, awareness and connectedness, balance, relaxation and healing.

Towards a Conclusion

Whilst the dominant Western metaphor of the body as machine is widely alluded to, the role of biology and biomedicine in symbolizing, indeed reifying, key cultural values in the West is less frequently acknowledged. Biomedical versions of anatomy, physiology and pathology permeate our society and our social sciences. The particular emphasis of Western medicine has only been possible since the beginning of the nineteenth century 'when ... biology emerged as a distinct subject and pathology became the basis of disease' (Armstrong 1987). Illich reminds us of the uniqueness (in time and, we might add, in place) of the extent of this influence:

We experienced a special moment in history when one agent, namely medicine, reached toward a monopoly over the social construction of bodily reality. (Illich 1986: 1325–6)

In some cases, the people I interviewed were questioning the very tenets of physiology, not as part of an ideological project, not as a deliberate challenge to biomedicine, but as part of a more pluralistic stance in relation to knowledge about their bodies. Whilst the notion of 'lay' knowledge is well established, it somehow carries with it, like a distinction between religious and lay orders, an implicit assumption of a superior authority of the non-lay group. Frankenberg (1994) has suggested that 'lay knowledge' is composed not just of different beliefs but constitutes a different kind of knowledge. If this is so, there may be a particular potency in the alliance of lay people/concepts and those alternative medicines which emphasize interconnectedness and the mobilizing of energy for healing.

The erosion of (some of) the cultural authority of biomedicine has been related by some (Bakx 1991) to a wider movement of disillusionment with the modernist project and of breakdown of key cultural institutions. Biomedical versions of anatomy, physiology and pathology have had a status which has been widely taken for granted; it is this status, perhaps, which is being re-negotiated. What is highlighted by the practitioners of Chi Kung is the process of interweaving different meanings and interpretations, again characterizing a key feature of a postmodern era (and place).[6] In this local instance at least, people are consciously recognizing a multiplicity of possibilities of knowing their bodies and their bodily suffering; among the cultural resources are various formal frameworks, and an acceptance of uncertainty is a necessary part of the interweaving of these. Whether talking about the biomedical approach or the traditional Chinese approach, knowledge is seen to be relative; claims to absolute knowing are refuted.

'I suppose I accept it [the idea of Chi] as a working hypothesis ... I think one just goes along with something that's workable, and I mean it's in the realm of philosophy, the absolute truth ... Like the theory of the atom, it's a workable theory, and so we go along with it.'

Acknowledgements

I am grateful to Ian Robinson and Ronnie Frankenberg for invaluable academic support during the genesis of this chapter, to Bob Skelton and Richenda Power for their perceptive comments on the draft, and to Helen Kent for providing me with a space in which to write it. Finally, my thanks go to Ursula Sharma and Sarah Cant for their insightful and sensitive editing.

Notes

1. I use the word 'consumer' rather reluctantly – see Stacey (1976) for some reservations on using the term in relation to health services – to indicate people who actually or potentially make use of alternative therapies/medicines.
2. I have used the terms 'alternative' practitioners here in preference to 'complementary'. The sense of being 'complementary' would be useful here if it were reciprocated by a recognition on the part of orthodox

medicine of its own complementary role. In using the term 'alternative', I imply a range of therapies and medicines which hold a non-official status.

3. There are both 'still' and cathartic styles of Chi Kung (Ots 1994); when I asked the teacher about this, he said that he preferred to leave people to discover any cathartic movements/experiences for themselves.

4. I have struggled – unsuccessfully – to find a useful term to denote my own ethnicity and that of the majority of my respondents, and have resorted to the generic term 'white'.

5. Whilst there are clearly significant differences between them, I use the terms 'the West'/'Western' as a shorthand for the geographical and social cluster of industrialized countries in Western Europe. I have extended Bourdieu's (1977) more culture specific habitus to the notion of a wider habitus.

6. Ed Soja has emphasized the significance of place in considering postmodernity, and Michael Rustin has questioned the ethnocentrism of a universalized category of postmodernism; with its notion of disruption of an earlier more stable modernity, it may hide the (human, economic, cultural) disruption associated with imperialism during the nineteenth and twentieth centuries. Comments were made at a session on Postmodern Spaces for a New Millennium at a conference on Postmodern Times at City University, London, 1995.

References

Armstrong, D. (1987) 'Bodies of Knowledge: Foucault and the Problem of Human Anatomy', in D. Scambler (ed.) Sociological Theory and Medical Sociology. London: Tavistock Publications.

Bakx, K. (1991) 'The Eclipse of Folk Medicine in Western Society'. Sociology of Health and Illness 13:1 21–38.

Benoist, J. and Cathebras, P. (1993) 'The Body: From an Immateriality to Another'. Social Science and Medicine 36(7): 857–65.

Bourdieu, P. (1977) Outline of a Theory of Practice, Richard Nice, trans. Cambridge: Cambridge University Press.

Crawford, R. (1985) 'A Cultural Account of "Health": Control, Release, and the Social Body', in J. McKinlay (ed.) Issues in the Political Economy of Health Care. London: Tavistock Publications.

Csordas, T. (1990) 'Embodiment as a Paradigm for Anthropology'. Ethos 18: 5–47.

Csordas, T. (1993) 'Somatic Modes of Attention'. Cultural Anthropology 8: 135–56.

Csordas, T. (ed.) (1994) Embodiment and Experience: The Existential Ground of Culture and Self. Cambridge: Cambridge University Press.

Douglas, M. (1994) 'The Construction of the Physician: A Cultural Approach to Medical Fashions', in S. Budd and U. Sharma (eds) The Healing Bond. London: Routledge.

Farquhar, J. (1991) 'Objects, Processes and Female Infertility in Chinese Medicine'. *Medical Anthropology Quarterly* 5: 4.

Frankenberg, R. (1994) 'What is Power? How is Decision? The Heart has its Reasons', in I. Robinson (ed.) *Life and Death under High Technology Medicine*. Manchester: Manchester University Press.

Geertz, C. (1973) 'Thick Description: Towards an Interpretive Theory of Culture', in C. Geertz, *The Interpretation of Cultures*. New York: Basic Books.

Gordon, D. (1988) 'Tenacious Assumptions in Western Medicine', in D. Gordon and M. Lock (eds) *Biomedicine Examined*. Dordrecht: Kluwer Academic Publishers.

Illich, I. (1986) 'Body History'. *Lancet* 2: 1325–7.

Kaptchuk, T. (1983) *Chinese Medicine: The Web that has no Weaver*. London: Century Hutchinson.

Kleinman *et al.* (1992) *Pain as Human Experience: An Anthropological Perspective*. Berkeley: University of California Press.

Martin, E. (1987) *The Woman in the Body*. Milton Keynes: Open University Press.

Okely, J. (1993) 'Participatory Experience and Embodied Knowledge', in J. Okely and H. Callaway (eds) *Anthropology and Autobiography*. London: Routledge.

Ots, T. (1994) 'The Silent Body – the Expressive Leib: On the Dialectic of Mind and Life in Chinese Cathartic Healing', in T. Csordas (ed.) *Embodiment and Experience: The Existential Ground of Culture and Self*. Cambridge: Cambridge University Press.

Pietroni, P. (1990) *The Greening of Medicine*. London: Gollancz.

Power, R. (1994) '"Only Nature Heals": A Discussion of Therapeutic Responsibility from a Naturopathic Point of View', in S. Budd and U. Sharma (eds) *The Healing Bond*. London: Routledge.

Sacks, O. (1984) *A Leg to Stand On*. New York: Harper and Row.

Saks, M. (ed.) 1992) *Alternative Medicine in Britain*. Oxford: Clarendon Press.

Scarry, E. (1985) *The Body in Pain: The Making and Unmaking of the World*. Oxford: Oxford University Press.

Stacey, M. (1976) 'The Health Service Consumer: A Sociological Misconception. Sociology of the NHS', *Sociology Review Monograph* 22. Keele: University of Keele.

7 Communicating the Individual Body and the Body Politic: The Discourse on Disease Prevention and Health Promotion in Alternative Therapies[1]

Espen Braathen

Introduction

This chapter is based upon a small-scale study in 1995 comprising extensive semi-structured interviews with twenty-five practitioners of homoeopathy working in the two largest cities of Norway, Oslo and Bergen. The aim of the study is to examine the perceptions and constructions of disease prevention and health promotion in alternative therapies, particularly within homoeopathy.

The chapter starts by introducing some central themes in the homoeopathic discourse on disease prevention and health promotion, paying particular attention to the construction of disease and the bodily expressions of symptoms. Health promotion is then discussed and defined within a comparative framework relating the homoeopathic ideas of health promotion to the conception of the phenomenon within the health promotion movement. The second part of the chapter is concerned with the relationship between the body and the body politic[2] and asks whether health promotion in homoeopathy is a new form of panoptic vision or rather a strategy for empowering the patient.

My point of departure feeds on the conviction that the current discourse in alternative therapies is intrinsically woven into a modernist version of the cultural dialogue between science and religion, knowledge and faith, scepticism and energistic or spiritual principles for constructing the world and the body. This discourse is, thus, part of an ongoing cultural struggle for defining the dominant forms and meanings of science and medicine.

Carol MacCormack, writing on the holistic health movement, contends that

> people in increasing numbers appear to be viewing themselves and all being within a framework of wholeness and implicate order. This is a world view in direct contrast to that of allopathic medicine which is based on a diagnostic process which splits people down to a diseased organ, and uses drugs which induce an opposite condition as part of the cure – to correct the malfunctioning part. (MacCormack 1991: 265)

The holistic health movement might be read as an embodied contestation of the ways in which people have come to see reality through a scientific world-view and, hence, a quest for living in a culture, to quote MacCormack again, 'which is simultaneously enriched by magic, religion and science, harmonised within a unified world view' (MacCormack 1991: 268).

The biological reductionism of biomedicine which tends to reduce the whole person to its biological body has become increasingly hard to accept wholeheartedly by most people (Benoist and Cathebras 1993). People tend to accept biological knowledge *per se* but they do not accept a purely biological conception of their own body. They conceive that there must be an immaterial part in the human body. This part, however, is not necessarily a supernatural one, but might be, as in the homoeopathic discourse, integral to nature.

Homoeopathy

The homoeopathic practitioners' narratives of disease prevention and health promotion are closely related to their dominant discourse of nature, wholeness and principles of the energistic body, all of which is spun around Hahnemann's axiom that 'all diseases are, in fact, diseases of the whole organism' (Hahnemann 1921). One homoeopath suggested to me that 'the use of homoeopathic remedies is also part of the process of restoring the balance of the remedy and, as such, homoeopathy is actually involved in healing the whole world'. Another homoeopath insisted that the remedies prescribed worked, according to not yet discovered natural laws, saying that 'it is important to allow nature itself to put things straight'. Nature is, in this context, to be understood as a physical reality, but one which is 'illuminated' by an omnipresent energy. The discourse on nature and the natural ways of curing becomes important in homoeopathy as nature and the individual body are seen as a whole, part and parcel of the same energistic organism.

Symptoms are, in the homoeopathic discourse, the natural *ur*-language of the body through which the disease 'talks' to the homoeopath. Because the disease, according to homoeopathic theory, is unknowable, its causes are known to man neither by the eye nor by the microscope. Hence, the body's symptomatology is the only way in which to express and respond to an underlying disturbance. 'Its response is', as Grossinger notes, 'actually a system-wide recognition of the existence of disease within itself and a synchronous attempt to allow the disease ... to express and vent itself with the least damage to the vital organs' (Grossinger 1980: 170).

The natural ways of curing, based upon Hahnemann's Law of Similars and Hering's Law,[3] also guide the homoeopathic discourse on disease prevention and health promotion. Before embarking on this issue it is necessary briefly to outline what is to be understood by these concepts.

Health Promotion and Homoeopathy

According to the tenets of the new public health movement[4] it is the effect of the total environment in health which is of concern, to the extent that socio-ecological and politico-economic issues seem to get the upper hand compared to individualized health-enhancing strategies. Don Nutbeam, writing from his position within the new public health establishment, defines disease prevention as representing 'strategies designed either to reduce risk-factors for specific disease, or to enhance host factors that reduce susceptibility to disease' (Nutbeam 1986: 115). Such strategies, focusing groups at risk and diseases, have been met with substantial critique, not least from medical anthropologists (Farmer 1992; Schiller 1992; 1994; Singer 1994), for blaming the victim and isolating disease-disposing factors from the wider socio-cultural environment contributing to health.

Health promotion, on the other hand, starts out with a vision of health as a resource for everyday life and focuses the whole population in the context of their daily activities. Thus, the World Health Organization (WHO) defines health promotion as 'the process of enabling people to increase control over, and to improve, their health' (WHO 1986). In order to carry out such an ambitious task health promotion actions work:

- to build healthy public policy;
- to create a supportive environment;
- to strengthen community action;
- to develop personal skills; and
- to reorient health services.

In sum, strategies which altogether stress the collective efforts to attain, maintain and reproduce health. Health promotion and disease prevention are frequently used synonymously but have to be seen as two separate, though complementary, strategies in the fight for public health (Chapman and Lupton 1994). This fight is, as Foucault (1984) has convincingly argued, fed by the modern state's preoccupation with controlling and shaping bodies.

Moving on to the homoeopathic discourse on these issues, it should become clear from the discussion which follows that this professional group of therapists share common ground with the health promotion movement. The homoeopathic view of disease prevention and health promotion is, as one would expect, solidly rooted in the therapeutic encounter and is, as such, basically an individualized strategy in which the individual body becomes the *locus nexus* for enhancing health.

As a leading homoeopath related to me: 'the homoeopathic interview is extremely important, and a solution to most problems is to be found here ... If the person had a better understanding of himself or herself this would radically improve the public health.' Societal or structural disease-disposing and health-enabling factors, and their importance, are not misconceived or denied by the homoeopaths, but as one homoeopath said to me: 'there is really nothing we can do at this level of causation'. Indeed, in the homoeopathic discourse, there is a widespread belief that these factors will, however, be reflected in the picture of symptoms which is always the endpoint of any therapeutic encounter and which the therapist and patient are obliged to work on in order to disclose.

It would be true to say that the homoeopaths have a clear, but rarely explicit, understanding and formulation of the structural constrains set by the body politic in matters concerning health. The homoeopathic line of argument emphasizes that the potentized remedy prescribed to the patient has the potential to effect processes of change which means that when the patient starts to get better he or she might go through an ontological transformation which has the power to alter the patient's relationship to both his or her individual body, as well as the social body. As one homoeopath told me: 'if the remedy hits the right strings it might revolutionize the patient's life'.

Cure and health promotion go hand in hand and, indeed, are inseparable as curative actions always have a preventive aim, namely to strengthen the patient's vital force to such an extent that the organism can rid itself of the problems that restrict the person. One homoeopath put it thus: 'Right treatment of a patient will always have a preventive effect. It strengthens the defence system in such a way as to enable the person to become less susceptible to disease.'

There is, however, another important, yet closely related thread running through the homoeopathic discourse which attests to homoeopaths' strong belief in raising the consciousness of the patient in matters of health and illness, and in particular in encouraging the patient to take responsibility for his or her own health. One homoeopath suggested that 'homoeopathy is a relatively cheap and simple form of cure but it does, indeed, demand active participation and commitment from the patient'. The issue of personal responsibility for health will be dealt with, but first I want to go back to what constitutes the common ground of homoeopathy and health promotion.

Both homoeopathy and health promotion share a deep scepticism of the biomedical model which is basically focused on disease and grounded in, what Gordon (1988) calls, some 'tenacious assumptions' concerning naturalism, individualism and reductionism which reproduces the dualistic thought system so deeply embedded in Western culture.

The focus on health, on the other hand, which characterizes the approach of homoeopathy and health promotion, celebrates health as a positive value, stressing its potential for achieving freedom and well-being.

Furthermore, they both pronounce disapproval of the harmful effects of medicine, and in particular the iatrogenic disturbances caused by over-medication. Empowerment or the process of enabling people to achieve their fullest health potential is also an important issue in both discourses.

Finally, emphasis is put on a holistic approach which is seen as essential for transcending the traditional biomedical model of disease and for realizing health. However, the issue of holism is also the line which divides the two camps. Wholeness in the homoeopathic discourse is limited to the individual body, although this body is perceived as a total energy complex comprising a mental-spiritual plane, an emotional-psychic plane, and a physical plane which all attach to the all-embracing organism of nature (Vithoulkas 1991).

Health promotion, on the other hand, adheres to the WHO's construction of wholeness as incorporating the physical, mental and social, thus paying attention to both the individual and the social body. There is, however, an emergent tendency in the health promotion discourse to account for the importance of the body politic, a focus which seems totally lacking in the homoeopathic discourse.

Health Promotion in Homoeopathy: Panoptic Vision ... ?

One of the most unexplained phenomena and least researched topic in the anthropology of alternative medicine is the relation between the body and the body politic which inevitably leads to the question of power and control. Anthropologist Ursula Sharma, for instance, discussing the therapeutic encounter and the differences between what happens in the consulting room of the GP and the homoeopath respectively, states that,

> to the extent that the complementary practitioner usually oper-ates quite independently of the state's interest in the bodies and health of its citizens there is always the potential for a very radical difference. Most complementary practice does not (at present) participate in the panoptical surveillance of citizens en-visaged by Foucault. (Sharma 1994: 102)

I would suggest that such a reading of Foucault is incomplete as his conception of disciplinary power, worked into subtle technolo-gies of the self, clearly points in the direction of harnessing bodies that are linked together in invisible relational networks and, as such, become unaware of its geometrical site of power and control.

Similarly, Norbert Elias (1939 [1994]) has suggested that power and power relations are interdependency ties intrinsic to the civiliz-ing process and the development of a body politic. It is interesting, with these perspectives in mind, to make a brief excursion into the highly relevant question of medicalization, understood as the pro-cess of labelling normal bodily functions and social issues as prob-lems requiring medical solutions.

Nancy Scheper-Hughes and Margaret Lock, writing on this topic, contend 'the usefulness to the body politic of filtering more and more human unrest, dissatisfaction, longing, and protest into the idiom of sickness, which can be safely managed by doctor-agents' (Scheper-Hughes and Lock 1987: 27). The stability of the body politic rests precisely on its ability to produce docile, though flexible, bodies, as Martin (1994) adds, conforming to the needs of the social and political order. Medicalization is thus a powerful strategy in which culturally specific definitions and meanings of health and social well-being are passed on and reproduced.

Homoeopaths oppose what they see as the medicalization of life and the hegemony of the doctor on the grounds that it deflects the person from understanding the wider mental-spiritual and emotional-psychic causes of health and robs the individuals of their responsibility for partaking in their own health development. Instead, they focus their gaze on health, promoting an option for gentleness (Douglas 1994) and personal responsibility for their own health. It would not be too far-fetched to suggest that the homoeopathic discourse constructs a new kind of medicalization through 'healthization' of life, as every aspect of the patient's life is of interest in establishing a complete symptom picture. This might be termed a new form of surveillance of life-worlds where the homoeopath, in contrast to the epidemiologically informed medico-social survey as an important device in the disciplining of populations, has become an important agent in carrying into effect self-disciplining technologies.

Technologies of the self are gentle in a political sense by procuring valuable information about the patient which is made unavailable for national health statistics but which strengthens the grip on private life-worlds and depoliticizes the work on health. The homoeopath is, moreover, in the therapeutic encounter and the work on the patient's health, consciously or unconsciously conveying powerful images of the current social and political order as a participant in a collective fight for public health.

In order to contextualize the dominant discourse on health in homoeopathy I will briefly discuss the heightened awareness and commercialization of health in consumer capitalism (Crawford 1984; Barsky 1988; Saltonstall 1993).

Ulrich Beck (1992) has developed the notion of the 'risk society' in which he points out the transformation that has taken place, due to modernization processes, with regard to the problem of risk. A general lesson imparted by his study refers to the fact that, as the natural causes of risks have been reduced, the man-made risks have dramatically increased in modern society. Accordingly, the consumer has been increasingly concerned with issues of risk and how to control or manage risks. Such a view is closely related to contemporary concerns with health issues, from the perspective of both the new public health and alternative therapies, as they all work on health in order to minimize the risks of diseases.

What distinguishes this gaze from the more traditional, biomedically based strategies of preventive medicine and public health is that bodies are now controlled under the new idiom of freedom and empowerment. Alternative therapies as well as the new public health movement also seem to invoke theories which are global, holistic, spiritual or ecological in scope compared to the local, partial and physical classification and theories of preventive medicine and public health. Furthermore, as consumption of commodities has become central to how people define themselves, the body and the work on health have come to be regarded as consumer commodities competing to maximize their market value.

Robert Crawford's study (1984) and Saltonstall's study (1993), almost a decade later, have examined the lay notions of health in the US population. Both studies underline the importance of self-control, discipline and deliberate, intentional actions in order to achieve health and improve one's bodily capital (Wacquant 1995). Crawford's (1984) study reinforces the critique launched in one of his earlier studies of the new health consciousness and movements (1980), where he examined how the construction of health in the holistic health movement and the self-care and self-help movements have been primarily concerned with a discourse on the individual body.

This discourse, which Crawford (1984) terms 'healthism', describing the belief or cultural value that health is the prime object of living, privatizes the struggle for societal well-being and thus reproduces, like the biomedical system, hegemonic values stressing individual responsibility for matters concerning health and disease.

... or Empowering Strategies?

In contrast to the disembodied discourse of preventive medicine and public health on health promotion, homoeopathy has located its discourse on the matter in the lives of its patients, evolving an embodied form of extraction of patients' data. As suggested, this constitutes a new kind of surveillance in which spiritual, psychological and emotional factors become increasingly important in a regime of discipline and regulation rather than the physical and social issues characterizing the medico-social survey.

However, this type of power/knowledge production is an ambiguous one. The nature of its dialectic, stressing the notion of personal responsibility for health, is at the same time the source of empowering strategies. Empowerment, defined as 'the notion of people having to take action to control and enhance their own lives, and the process of enabling them to do so' (Grace 1991: 330), has become the dominant aim and symbol of health-promoting strategies. What the homoeopaths are doing both in the therapeutic encounter and by prescribing remedies are in fact perceived as empowering actions. As one homoeopath put it: 'We (the homoeopaths) must help the patient to a fuller and more adequate life'; or another example: 'homoeoepathy contributes to a harmonious development of the person in his or her own surroundings'.

The 'optical' image that Sharma (1994) is referring to – the homoeopath seeing himself or herself as a mirror reflecting back an image of the patient's life – represents a metaphor of the Law of Similars which I often came across in my interviews. The invocation of reactions in the patient's body during the therapeutic encounter that are similar to his or her symptoms is rendered vital, however difficult, in fuelling the healing process. The therapist has, thus, an essential role in enabling the patient to take control and enhance his or her own life and health.

Conclusion

Throughout the chapter it has been an explicit aim to examine how power and control necessarily have to be an important issue in the discourse on health promotion in homoeopathy. The dialectic of this discourse clearly shows how the production of power/knowledge in homoeopathy is a balance between the surveillance and regulation of citizens, and promoting empowering strategies for enhancing health.

The individualized strategy of empowerment in homoeopathy pays limited attention to the social and, indeed, politico-economic determinants necessary for facilitating changes influencing the factors which restrict the person. The homoeopathic strategies of empowering the patient are firmly rooted in the therapeutic encounter and the prescription of remedies. The therapeutic encounter and prescription of remedies are fundamental to the homoeopathic understanding of the potentials as well as the limitations of homoeopathic interventions. The homoeopathic contribution to improving the public health is basically through individualized actions in which each person's individual symptom picture is the key to cure and attaining health.

In conclusion, it is indeed worth noticing the way in which the medical gaze of homoeopathy is directed. As the physical examination of the patient plays only a very limited role in the homoeopathic therapeutic encounter, the making of the body takes a somewhat different direction from that described by Foucault (1976). According to Foucault, the medical body was made into a static object which could be explored and examined according to the spatialization of its surface dimensions, its anatomy and its social space. The homoeopathic discourse constructs an energistic body; a living, flexible organism which adapts and responds to its environment. Its responses can be read through the body's production of symptoms. To promote health the homoeopath prescribes potentized homoeopathic remedies in order to invoke the individual body's self-healing energies.

Notes

1. This paper was presented at the third International Network for Research on Alternative Therapies (INRAT) seminar in Denmark, Værløse 29 September – 1 October 1995. It will be published in: Helle Johannessen et al. (eds) Studies in Alternative Therapy 3, Odense: Odense University Press, 1996. Thanks to the participants in the section on 'Communicating in and about the body', for their helpful comments and to Odense University Press, with whose kind permission it is reproduced here.

2. The body politic refers to the third level of Scheper-Hughes and Lock's (1987) conceptualization of the three bodies: the individual body, the social body and the body politic, respectively. The latter concerns the issues of power and control in the relationships between individual and social bodies. According to Scheper-Hughes and Lock, 'an anthropology of relations between the body and the body politic inevitably leads to a consideration of the regulation and control not only of individuals but of populations' (Scheper-Hughes and Lock 1987: 27).

3. Hering's Law refers to the influential work of Hahnemann's follower Constantine Hering who developed notions about the specific order of curative sequences in homoeopathy. According to Hering a cure proceeds from above downwards and from within outwards. Furthermore, when a cure is in progress the symptoms disappear in the reverse order of their coming (in Ullman 1988).

4. The new public health movement emerged in the 1970s and was a response to the preoccupation with individual health more generally of the twentieth century. The new public health movement wants to

regenerate the original public health movement of the nineteenth century and its focus of interventions at environmental infrastructures affecting health (Bunton and Macdonald 1992). Deborah Lupton contends that the history of 'the "new" public health is typically represented as a reaction against both the individualistic and victim blaming approach of health education and the curative model of biomedicine. It is heralded as a return to the concern with environmental factors that first generated the public health movement of the nineteenth century. ... Health promotion is a central plank of the "new" public health' (Lupton 1995: 50).

References

Beck, U. (1992) Risk Society. Towards a New Modernity. Sage: London.
Barsky, A. J. (1988) 'The Paradox of Health'. The New England Journal of Medicine, 318(7): 414–18.
Benoist, J. and Cathebras, P. (1993) 'The Body: From an Immateriality to Another. Social Science and Medicine, 36(7): 857–65.
Bunton, R. and Macdonald, G. (1992) 'Health Promotion: Discipline or Disciplines?', in R. Bunton and G. Macdonald (eds) Health Promotion: Disciplines and Diversity. Routledge: London.
Chapman, S. and Lupton, D. (1994) 'The Fight for Public Health. Principles and Practice of Media Advocacy'. British Medical Journal. London: Publishing Group.
Crawford, R. (1980) 'Healthism and the Medicalization of Everyday Life'. International Journal of Health Services, 10(3): 365–88.
Crawford, R. (1984) 'A Cultural Account of "Health": Control, Release, and the Social Body', in J. B. McKinlay (ed.) Issues in the Political Economy of Health Care. London: Tavistock, pp. 61–103.
Douglas, M. (1994) 'The Construction of the Physician: A Cultural Approach to Medical Fashion', in S. Budd and U. Sharma (eds) The Healing Bond. The Patient–Practitioner Relationship and Therapeutic Responsibility. London: Routledge, pp. 23–41.
Elias, N. (1939 [1994]) The Civilizing Process. Blackwell: Oxford.
Farmer, P. (1992) AIDS and Accusation. Haiti and the Geography of Blame. Berkeley: University of California Press.
Foucault, M. (1976) The Birth of the Clinic: An Archaeology of Medical Perception. London: Tavistock.
Foucault, M. (1984) 'The Politics of Health in the Eighteenth Century', in P. Rabinow (ed.) The Foucault Reader. London: Penguin.
Gordon, D. (1988) 'Tenacious Assumptions in Western Medicine', in M. Lock and D. Gordon (eds) Biomedicine Examined. Dordrecht: Kluwer Academic Publishers.
Grace, V. M. (1991) 'The Marketing of Empowerment and the Construction of the Health Consumer: A Critique of Health Promotion', International Journal of Health Services 21(2): 329–43.

Grossinger, R. (1980) *Planet Medicine. From Stone Age Shamanism to Post-Industrial Healing.* London: Shambhale.

Hahnemann, S. (1991/2) *Organon of Medicine.* Berkeley: North Atlantic Books.

Lupton, D. (1995) *The Imperative of Health. Public Health and the Regulated Body.* London: Sage.

MacCormac, C. P. (1991) 'Holistic Health and a Changing Western World View', *Curare* 7: 259–73.

Martin, E. (1994) *Flexible Bodies. Tracking Immunity in American Culture from the Days of Polio to the Age of AIDS.* Boston: Beacon Press.

Nutbeam, D. (1986) 'Health Promotion Glossary'. *Health Promotion* 1(1): 113–27.

Saltonstall, R. (1993) 'Healthy Bodies, Social Bodies: Men's and Women's Concepts and Practices of Health in Everyday Life'. *Social Science and Medicine* 36(1): 7–14.

Scheper-Hughes, N. and Lock, M. M. (1987) 'The Mindful Body: A Prolegomenon to Future Work in Medical Anthropology'. *Medical Anthropology Quarterly* 1(1): 6–41.

Schiller, N. G. (1992) 'What's Wrong With This Picture? The Hegemonic Construction of Culture in AIDS Research in the United States'. *Medical Anthropology Quarterly* 6(3): 237–45.

Schiller, N. G. (1994) 'Risky Business: The Cultural Construction of AIDS Risk Groups'. *Social Science and Medicine* 38(10): 1337–46.

Sharma, U. (1994) 'The Equation of Responsibility: Complementary Practitioners and Their Patients' in S. Budd and U. Sharma (eds) *The Healing Bond. The Patient–Practitioner Relationship and the Therapeutic Responsibility.* London: Routledge.

Singer, M. (1994) 'AIDS and the Health Crisis of the U.S. Urban Poor: The Perspective of Critical Medical Anthropology'. *Social Science and Medicine,* 39(7): 931–48.

Ullman, D. (1988) *Discovering Homoeopathy. Medicine for the 21st Century.* Berkeley: North Atlantic Books.

Vithoulkas, G. (1991) *A New Model of Health and Disease.* Berkeley: North Atlantic Books.

Wacquant, L. J. D. (1995) 'Pugs at Work: Bodily Capital and Bodily Labour Among Professional Bxers'. *Body and Society* 1(1): 65–93.

World Health Organization (1986) *The Ottawa Charter for Health Promotion.* Ottawa/Copenhagen: WHO.

PART FOUR

Situating Medical Knowledge

Codifying selected knowledge and engaging with the scientific medical paradigm for the purpose of public legitimation (as discussed in the first section in this book) is not the only way in which complementary practitioners attempt to ground and comprehend their knowledge systems. It is also possible to situate therapeutic knowledge more informally and in relation to non-medical ways of knowing.

Ursula Sharma's study shows the variety of mapping practices undertaken by homoeopaths to situate their knowledge. Interested homoeopaths have made links to (for example) Jungian psychology, to tie what they know about their practice to other forms of cultural knowledge. This contributes to the grounding of homoeopathic knowledge by suggesting new (non-medical) ways of understanding how homoeopathy works, as well as reflecting the individual backgrounds and interests of practitioners. This situating work, and the debates it engenders, is best understood as part of the process of consolidating knowledge internal to the profession and is rarely employed to elicit external legitimacy.

8 Situating Homoeopathic Knowledge: Legitimation and the Cultural Landscape

Ursula Sharma

Professional knowledge has a paradoxical aspect. On the one hand, it is restricted, even mysterious. For a profession to maintain any kind of privileged niche, access to these mysteries must be jealously guarded. Not for nothing have sociologists of the professions stressed processes of closure (Crompton 1987). On the other hand, the process of obtaining such a privileged niche must also involve convincing those outside the profession that its knowledge is valid and useful, actually necessary to society. However we characterize the process of legitimation, it is bound to involve some exposure to scrutiny of the knowledge claims of the professionalizing group. Public accountability is incompatible with total secrecy.

Where groups of complementary therapists have (with varying degrees of success) attempted to gain professional status in Britain and other European countries, this scrutiny of their knowledge has been of three kinds.

First, there is the scrutiny of the state. If the state is to license practitioners, then the legislators must be convinced that the claims of the practitioners are valid, that what they claim to do is not only useful and therefore worth licensing, but that they really can do it, that their claims to special knowledge do have some basis.

Second, in practice this has also meant convincing members of the orthodox medical profession, to the extent that the legislators have relied heavily (though not exclusively) on the advice and dispositions of this profession in matters concerning the registration of health care practitioners.

Third, the claims to knowledge of a professional group must be supported to some extent by the public at large. However much it may convince itself of its own autonomy and self-containment, however self-referential its rhetoric, a profession or discipline also 'addresses' the public; in the end it needs to 'legitimate its existence vis-à-vis other disciplines and society at large' (Robbins 1993: 116). The notion of 'public' is a very vague and heterogeneous concept and I use it here only as a shorthand way of referring to the fact that it is not only the state and the medical profession with whom complementary practitioners' knowledge claims must carry conviction. There must be a widespread (though not necessarily universal) cultural acceptance of the validity of the claims to professional knowledge and practice of the group concerned. There must be some kind of trust that the form of professional knowledge in question can be mapped on to other forms of knowledge in society. These links may remain ambiguous and less than explicit or fully worked out so far as the individual potential user of the group's professional services is concerned. The detailed working out of this cultural legitimation can, after all, be left to the 'experts'.

On the whole, social scientists who have studied complementary therapies have concerned themselves mainly with the second level of legitimation; specifically with the relationship between complementary medicines and the orthodox medical profession. They have even tended to define their field, and the problems within it, in terms of complementary medicines' lack of scientific medical endorsement, their failure to relate to current medical orthodoxies (Wallis and Morley 1976). This was quite reasonable since complementary therapists themselves long regarded the persuasion of the medical profession as their main political problem. Indeed some fascinating work has resulted from sociologists' exploration of the politics of the interface between alternative medical systems and of knowledge and orthodox medicine itself (Nicholls 1988; Saks 1995). However, the understandable emphasis on the rejection of these forms of knowledge by the medical profession, as 'illegitimate' or 'marginal' knowledge, and so on, has tended to stress their intellectual isolation, and has focused on cultural discontinuity rather than continuity.

In this chapter I wish to look at some of the ways in which a group of homoeopaths have traced relationships between their own and other bodies of knowledge, the process of 'situating' their knowledge in a broader cultural landscape. Much of the 'situating' work I shall describe in this chapter was not performed by way of intentional apologia or with the conscious aim of persuading the public (indeed much of it appears in house journals circulated mainly within the profession). Rather it can be understood as a way in which reflective members of the professional group build constructive links between different bodies of knowledge with which they are familiar, thus 'de-isolating' their professional knowledge, 'de-marginalizing' it.

Cultural legitimation, the rather diffuse process by which members of a profession affirm the consistency of their professional knowledge with other publicly valued forms of knowledge, does not only therefore involve rhetoric aimed at the general public. It may also involve the *intra*-professional discourses by which members of the profession affirm *to each other* the situatedness of their professional knowledge and suggest to one another the kind of links which are relevant or might be appropriately pursued, what other bodies of knowledge may provide inspiration.

There may be disagreement as to which connections are best pursued, and this kind of uncertainty is precisely what we would expect if we accept that we are seeing a crisis of legitimation in the sense that Lyotard described. If it is true that science has experienced an erosion of the foundations of its claim to legitimacy so that there is a 'loosening of the encyclopaedic net in which each science was to find itself' (Lyotard 1986: 39), then homoeopaths may well find themselves uncertain as to how to respond to demands that they prove their knowledge to be 'scientific', unsure as to which form of science (if any) they should claim kinship with, what place their knowledge might take in a rapidly disintegrating nexus. On the basis of a discussion of the way in which homoeopaths have engaged in a broader cultural legitimation of their knowledge, I shall offer some more general theoretical observations on the fragmentation and unity of cultural knowledge.

The professional community with which I am concerned is the Society of Homoeopaths, and it is the writings of their members which I shall draw upon here, as well as my own observations at their conferences and meetings, and some interviews carried out with members.[1] The Society of Homoeopaths is the larger of two groups of non-medically qualified (hereafter NMQ) homoeopaths in Britain, having about 360 licensed members (see Cant, in this volume). Whilst this group has its own specific features and its own intellectual atmosphere, some of the legitimation problems it has experienced are shared by other groups of homoeopaths in some form or another. Let us start therefore with some observations on the form and organization of homoeopathic knowledge in general.

Codifying Homoeopathic Knowledge: Science, Riddles and Indeterminancies

Homoeopathy as a healing modality was founded by Samuel Hahnemann (1755–1843). The fundamental principle which Hahnemann established was that 'like cures like', that is, disease is best cured by the administration of a substance which, in its natural form, produces symptoms the same as or similar to those from which the patient suffers. However, these substances are not administered in their 'raw' form (some of those used in homoeopathic practice are, in their naturally occurring state, highly toxic) but in an extremely dilute form, 'potentized' by a process of vigorous vibration or 'succussion'. Various degrees of dilution are used, some of them so high that a given dose may contain no molecules of the original substance at all.

The distinctiveness of homoeopathy, however, does not lie solely in the kind of medicines it uses, but also in its nosology. One could even say that it has no nosology, for homoeopathy interprets the symptoms from which the patient complains less in terms of named 'diseases' than in terms of the constitution of the patient. The homoeopath attempts to elicit a profile of the patient which will include not just his or her current pathology, but general tendencies and proclivities such as tastes for certain kinds of food, emotional temperament, and so on, which would not in other contexts necessarily be considered in terms of 'symptoms'. Much (though not all) homoeopathic prescribing consists of the attempt to find the remedy whose profile (in terms of its known effects) best matches the constitutional profile of the patient: 'that substance which is similar to the totality of symptoms, spiritual, mental, emotional and physical, of our patient' (Wright Hubbard 1990: 7).

Common to most homoeopathic practice is the idea that 'less means more' – the smaller the dose, the greater the potential effect on the patient (provided that the remedy has been properly potentized and correctly prescribed). This, of course, flies in the face of both scientific and everyday common sense. In pharmaceutical terms *more* substance need not always mean *more* effects (the body may stop absorbing a substance prescribed over a certain limit and simply eliminate it), but *less* cannot possibly mean *more*. And a substance which may not even be present in a given dose (as in the case of very high dilutions) cannot possibly exert any effect on the patient, beneficial or otherwise.

Hahnemann did not offer any coherent theory as to exactly how or why homoeopathically prepared remedies affect the patient. He proposed that there must be some non-corporeal energy at work which we do not have to understand fully in order to harness for the benefit of patients (Hahnemann 1986: 101). There is therefore a riddle at the heart of homoeopathic knowledge.

There have, it is true, been some recent attempts to subject the theory of the action of the microdose to testing through laboratory experiments, the most famous being that of Benveniste (Poitevin *et al.* 1988). And homoeopaths themselves have certainly theorized about the nature of whatever force allows 'less' to produce 'more' (for example, Vithoulkas 1980). But most homoeopaths seem able to accept what I have called the 'riddle' at the heart of homoeopathy as a problem that may one day be solved by scientific investigation, as a paradox which they are prepared for the time being to accept. From the point of view of the public, both scientifically educated and otherwise, therefore, homoeopathy not only flies in the face of common sense, but it seems quite content to continue to operate with this riddle unsolved.

There is another less salient problem. Professionalization involves the consolidation and systematization of knowledge, its codification so that it can be transmitted through accepted and certified forms of professional education. A college curriculum based on an acknowledged mystery or riddle such as the one just discussed may be hard to justify. Yet some homoeopathic knowledge is hard to codify for quite different reasons. Whilst Hahnemann and his successors were quite capable of formulating some general principles or even 'laws' in the form of general propositions about the ways in which homoeopathic treatment works, the acceptance of the infinite variability of the human organism, the stress on the specific constitution of the patient, means that treatments of actual cases are based on very *local* forms of knowledge. This consists of the information which the patient and the practitioner can put together between them about the patient's propensities and state of health. Individuals only approximately conform to constitutional types, and constitutional types themselves are not closed and determinate.

Looking at the issue from another angle, knowledge of remedies themselves is open ended. One important way in which homoeopathic knowledge is expanded is through the kind of experimentation which Hahnemann called a 'proving', in which the effects of a new remedy are explored through its administration to a sample of healthy adults. Whilst a homoeopath who organizes a proving hopes to collect data on as many of the effects of the remedy as s/he possibly can, the effect of the remedy on the organism is also not fixed and determinate. A good homoeopath can in principle always find more applications of a remedy, more characteristics of the type to which it corresponds, even if in practice most homoeopaths work with only a few of the indications recorded in the materia medica for a given remedy. Thus we find that much knowledge among NMQ homoeopaths is transmitted in terms of 'I found that ...', or 'in my experience ...'. Seminars are often the transmission of *experience* rather than readily codified knowledge.

From these remarks it is easy to understand why many NMQ homoeopaths do not see the relevance of the type of trial preferred by the medical scientist for a new medical intervention or pharmaceutical product. The randomized clinical trial is designed to produce generalizable knowledge about the standardized effects of a particular intervention which (ideally at least) can be regarded as true of all populations at all times, the antithesis of the local knowledge of a specific body with all its individual peculiarities.

To summarize what has been said so far, we can see that homoeopaths will have specific problems in situating their knowledge in relation to medical and physical science so long as these constitute dominant forms of knowledge. More generally, homoeopaths are likely to have problems in converting the highly specific and practical everyday knowledge of practitioners (based in part on local knowledge of patients' bodies and experiences) into codified knowledge which non-homoeopaths can recognize as a culturally valid form of knowledge. If homoeopathy is not a form of scientific knowledge, as popularly understood, what other kind of knowledge might it be and what other kind of legitimacy might it have?

For doctor homoeopaths, trained by the Faculty of Homoeopaths, there is already a degree of commitment to medical science and for them a major problem is trying to locate homoeopathic knowledge in relation to this corpus of knowledge. The issue of whether or not homoeopathy is scientific, which has been hotly debated from time to time among medical homoeopaths (see Campbell 1978; Fisher 1981) turns out to be very much a problem about how to represent homoeopathy to non-homoeopath medical colleagues within the profession (see particularly Campbell 1978: 84).

For NMQ homoeopaths the issues are somewhat different. They, too, debate the issue of the scientificity of homoeopathy in general, but are less concerned with its relationship to medical science in particular. They do not, after all, have any particular commitment to or detailed familiarity with this body of knowledge, even though they share a concern that homoeopathy be accepted as a legitimate form of treatment by the medical profession in general. But, as we shall see, they are perhaps more comfortable with the 'Janus faced' nature of homoeopathy (Campbell 1984), the way in which it faces both the empirical and rationalistic tradition of therapeutics of which modern medicine is a major manifestation, but also a metaphysical tradition of thinking about the human person. The issue of the scientificity of homoeopathy is certainly debated, but with greater acceptance that homoeopathy could be situated both within a scientific tradition of thought and within other important traditions. The title of the eleventh annual conference of the Society of Homoeopaths made witty reference to this tension or ambivalence; 'HeART and SciENCE'. The conference was billed as combining 'new dimensions of fact and feeling'.

Homoeopathy and (What Sort of) Science?

One response of NMQ homoeopaths has been to suggest that there is no need for homoeopathy to reject science as such, but that there is no room for it within conventional pre-quantum science.

Complementary therapists seeking to relate their knowledge to the prestigious knowledge of the natural sciences have not been slow to pick up on debates about epistemology, especially debates about the nature of science and the recent questioning of the idea that natural scientific knowledge constitutes a totally objective body of knowledge established once and for all, independent of context, especially social context. Kuhn's notion of the scientific paradigm is referred to frequently. Amir Cassam, for instance, wrote an article entitled 'Need homoeopathy be a science?' in *The Homoeopath* in which he argues that

> Homoeopathy ... represents a new 'paradigm' with its own new rationality which has come about not by a process of accretion to the gradually built up core of medical 'scientific' knowledge but as a revolutionary break from it. Indeed, that is how science develops in all fields. (Cassam 1994: 240)

He makes approving reference to Feyerabend's propositions that there is not a single method in science that is absolutely binding, and that major developments in knowledge occur just because the currently accepted rules have been violated. One might also point to an article in *The Homoeopath* on models of research, in which the author refers disparagingly to positivist paradigms and approvingly to William James's notion of 'radical empiricism' in which subjective experience is not ruled out as a form of data (Wansborough 1995).

One line of discussion which we find in this community of therapists is the idea that whilst the 'riddle' referred to above is a problem within conventional Newtonian physics, it may not be a problem within other paradigms. There is thus much reference to quantum physics, and to the work of Capra. In a widely read book, *The Science of Homoeopathy*, the famous Greek homoeopath Vithoulkas quotes extensively from *The Tao of Physics*. If matter and energy are interchangeable, what I have called the riddle at the centre of homoeopathy is not a riddle at all, or constitutes a very different kind of riddle, and Vithoulkas argues that

homoeopathy, in comparison to orthodox medicine, has – on therapeutic grounds – the same difference that quantum mechanics bears to Newtonian physics. It was obvious that after the entrance of homoeopathy into the therapeutic field, the physician was able to affect, in a curative way, through the energized homoeopathic remedy, the electromagnetic field of the patient. (Vithoulkas 1980: xvi)

One might regard the kind of discourse quoted above as the very selective use of scientific ideas on the part of people who have little deep understanding of modern scientific knowledge in order to provide support for a particular position. Probably most NMQ homoeopaths are people with a non-scientific background. Yet some have formerly pursued careers in pharmacy, engineering and other disciplines requiring a knowledge of some branch or other of natural science. Amir Cassam, whom I quoted above, is a trained dentist. Jazz Rasool is a researcher in crystallography at London University who also teaches physics at the London College of Classical Homoeopathy. In an article in *The Homoeopath*, he refers to holistic theories of the universe and discusses the idea of the homoeopathic remedy resonating with the frequency of an illness in terms of the operation of electromagnetic fields, with much reference to Einstein, Schrödinger, Von Neumann, among others (Rasool 1994: 209). Such discourse cannot be dismissed as superficial uninformed apologetics.

Classification as an Intellectual Bridge: The Periodic Table and the Doctrine of Signatures

A number of homoeopaths have engaged with quite specific bodies of scientific knowledge outside physics. The idea of constitutional types lends itself to linkage with other classificatory sets, series, lists, types, and so on, and this has facilitated the tracking of linkage with other bodies of knowledge. This, as we shall see, allows for a more creative and flexible use of other bodies of knowledge, pursuing what are in effect relations of analogy rather than relations of substantive consistency.

One example of this is the fascination which the periodic table currently holds for a number of prominent homoeopaths in the Society. This was a theme touched on in a number of presentations and discussions at the 1992 and 1993 annual conferences, possibly stimulated by the famous Indian homoeopath Rajan Sankaran's known interest in the subject. According to an article by Helen Holt (trained as a chemist before she became a homoeopath), this interest goes back to the 1930s when Otto Leeser first suggested that the periodic table might provide an aid to studying elements considered as remedies, and their similarities (Holt 1994). Holt's discussion of the periodic table is characteristic of this discourse in that she tries to relate the properties of the elements, as understood by chemists, to the properties of the remedies derived from these elements, as understood by homoeopaths. To give an example, she points out that the characteristic of group VII, the halogens, is their 'energy':

> Iodine is an interesting solid – when heated it does not let into a liquid but turns straight into a gas, producing clouds of violet vapour (chemists say that it 'sublimes' – only one other element sublimes on heating, and that is carbon in the form of graphite) ...
>
> So with all the energy present in these elements, it is not surprising this is reflected in their properties as homoeopathic remedies. Scholten summed it up when he described the keynotes of these elements – he described Fluoratum compounds as being hard, fast and hurried; Bromatums have a desire to escape – they are restless and fond of travelling. (Holt 1994: 267)

An article by Mike Andrews in the same edition of *The Homoeopath* suggests that we would expect the elements (1–30 and 53) which occur naturally in the human body to be more often indicated as remedies. However,

> the heavier elements are less frequently indicated, and indicative of a more severe pathology. In terms of what they have done to the balance of the planet they are obviously increasingly indicated. Heavy metals have entered the food chain! (Andrews 1994: 243)

This interest in the periodic table has actually stimulated some new provings, notably Jeremy Sherr's (1992) proving of hydrogen. It would be impossible to summarize his observations on the results of the proving, but as a sample of the kind of relationships he traces between the properties of hydrogen (considered from the point of view of the chemist) and the properties of potentized hydrogen revealed in the proving, we note that provers recorded feelings such as 'a feeling of being pulled downwards' which Sherr relates to the process of birth, 'just as hydrogen gave birth to the pattern of all the other elements in the Periodic Table' (Sherr 1992).

The structure of this kind of discourse is reminiscent of another (on the face of it, quite different) way of relating remedy to nature which recurs in homoeopathic discussions, namely appeal to some version of the doctrine of signatures. In an address given at the 1992 conference, later published as an article, Dana Ullman reminds us that

> the doctrine of signatures is an ancient concept that assumed that a plant was good for healing that which it looked like. The plant Great Celandine was yellow and thus it was good for the liver and the yellow bile it created. (Ullman 1993: 27)

This theory, he argues, was a very crude theory but, nonetheless, the exploration of what biologists know about natural species can give us hints about the use of remedies derived from these species, and he makes a case for

> studying how the substances we use in homoeopathy exist and act in nature as a way to get reliable and insightful information about when to prescribe them. (Ullman 1993: 27)

One of the examples he gives is the remedy Sepia, derived from the ink of the cuttlefish. Among the properties of the cuttlefish is its capacity to change colour to mimic its surroundings.

The sepia person's ability to change colours is typified by his or her tendency to seem kind and friendly but change into being argumentative, obstinate and narrow-minded. Many women who need sepia develop male traits in the business world, changing their own colours by suppressing their femininity. (Ullman 1993: 29).

Another example is colocynthis, a member of the cucurbit family of plants, whose bristly stem and prickly leaves relate to an 'irritable unsociable nature' from which homoeopathic doses of colocynthis can offer relief.

In a commentary on the 1994 conference of the Society, Jerome Whitney reflected on this recurrence of analogue and classification, remarking that a theme that might be said to unify the various discussions in the conference was that of alchemy.

Throughout the conference alchemy permeated and riveted our attention, as an example the representation on plants using the Doctrine of Sign, Signature and Simillimum aiding our understanding of the remedies. However this was not done in a simplistic way; yellow is for liver complaints; but in the more clear, technical and useful ways. In a lucid lecture on Sunday evening the alchemical classification of the qualities of the four kingdoms, mineral, vegetable, animal and human, emerged as a powerful way to relate to the quality, manner and ambience of the patient in order to aid in the designation of the kingdom from which the remedy could be chosen. (Whitney 1994: 23)

If not Rationalism, Then What?

The Paracelsan influence on homoeopathy, which Jerome Whitney refers to, is something of which homoeopaths are keenly aware. A dominant theme in discussion and publications of the Society is the need to integrate the rationalism of modern science without discarding the philosophical underpinnings of homoeopathy, even if Swedenborgianism and the other various more metaphysical traditions which have animated groups of homoeopaths at various times are not publicly reclaimed by the collectivity. The Society of Homoeopaths grew from foundations laid by the pupils of two charismatic teachers, Da Monte and Maughan (see Cant, in this volume) who were self-confessed Druids and evidently, according to the testimony of their pupils, saw homoeopathy as a means to spiritual development, not just the cure of symptoms. The Society of Homoeopaths as a collectivity has chosen to move away from any explicit association of homoeopathy with such doctrines, although many individual homoeopaths see the connection between homoeopathy and spiritual development as crucial to their personal practice of the therapy.

A direction which some homoeopaths have taken which obviates some of the problems and unease which the dilemma of rationalism potentially involves is to relate homoeopathic knowledge more closely to psychotherapeutic knowledge. This direction allows the homoeopath to explore the emotional and spiritual dimension of the individual whilst referring to a body of knowledge which is regarded as being in some way (albeit tenuously by many) grounded in empirical knowledge of human beings. A very influential homoeopath working in this tradition is Edward Whitmont who is also a Jungian analyst. The use of a basically Jungian framework allows the homoeopath to refer to archetypes, myths and symbols, yet in a way that distances the therapist from literal belief in mythological personages such as Hecate, the Goddess. Lisa Chera tells us, for instance, that the symbolic content of dreams needs to be decoded, but with due consciousness of the ways in which female archetypes have been distorted by patriarchal influences in history (Chera 1994: 330).

Elisabeth Danciger, in a discussion of the 'wounded healer', explores the various images of suffering available in the Western mythological fund (the Fisher King, the Hanged Man of the Tarot, the story of Chiron, and so on) in order to understand better the ways in which the healer uses his or her own woundedness to empathize with the patient: 'Symbolic stories are a great gift for they continually open up new ways of seeing, perceiving and experiencing our realities' (Danciger 1993: 132).

Here homoeopathic understanding is related to a body of cultural knowledge other than the natural sciences, a tradition which permits more reference to history and social process. It is more sophisticated and probably more widely credible than, for example, Vannier's attempts to relate homoeopathic remedies to types and prototypes derived from Graeco-Roman mythology – the Marsian type, the Mercurian type, and so on (Vannier 1992). It is a kind of situating work which will succeed better in an age where people derive their knowledge of mythology less from direct readings of the ancient classics themselves and more from the works of therapists like Jung himself, or from the derivative mythologies of New Age ideas and practices.

Some General Features of 'Situating' Work:
The Limits of Eclecticism

Homoeopaths, as we have seen, do not operate in a cultural vacuum but attempt to situate their therapeutic knowledge in relation to other bodies of knowledge. But perhaps this web of linkages grows somewhat too dense. Can one really relate homoeopathic knowledge to bodies of knowledge as diverse as Jungian archetypes and the periodic table? Extreme eclecticism may surely undermine attempts to legitimize professional knowledge. It may expose the profession to ridicule from without, and encourage excessive heterogeneity of approach from within. At the collective level, surely choices may have to be made, some intellectual connections repudiated and others brought to the fore?

Whilst some have commented with satisfaction on the ways in which modern homoeopathy seems able to integrate both a scientific and spiritual approach to healing, others have noted the tensions in the web of connections I have described. I have already referred to Campbell's depiction of homoeopathy as 'Janus faced', and some might identify the kind of 'situating' work I have been describing in terms of a dualistic split rather than a criss-crossing web of constructive connections.

Thus Denis MacEoin, in an article which fired considerable controversy within the Society, argued that it matters a great deal whether homoeopaths seek to link their knowledge and practice with the empirical rationalist tradition of natural scientific enquiry or with what he regards as the more esoteric traditions favoured by some homoeopaths (alchemy, astrology, archetypes, New Age ideas; not to mention the Druidism of the teachers of the original founders of the Society). As far as the *patient* is concerned, MacEoin argues, one cannot have one's cake and eat it. The integration of homoeopathy with the most advanced scientific ideas claimed by some may not be self-evident to the patient who, on the contrary, may in the consulting room encounter an alienating homoeopathy apparently informed by ideas which he or she regards as bunkum or 'esoteric dogma' (MacEoin 1993: 113).

There is much more to MacEoin's argument than this, but I cite his article to indicate that, whilst the output of the Society suggests intellectual eclecticism and a willingness to find connections between homoeopathy and a variety of other bodies of knowledge, there may be practical and political limitations to such collective eclecticism, especially considered in terms of the process of legitimation in the eyes of the public, which I mentioned earlier. There are already existing discontinuities in the cultural field within which homoeopathy places itself which cannot be overlooked, and possibly a group cannot link its knowledge successfully to all the different kinds of cultural knowledge without incurring certain practical costs.

Concluding Discussion:
Webs, Lattices and Landscapes

In this chapter I have discussed some of the ways in which an emerging professional group of homoeopaths have attempted to link their own specialized knowledge to other bodies of cultural knowledge. As one might expect, the relationship between homoeopathic knowledge to 'science' is a major preoccupation, but science is by no means the only body of knowledge with which homoeopaths have sought connections.

I presented this tracing of linkages initially in terms of a process of cultural legitimation. This cultural process is not, of course, unrelated to the political processes by which some groups of healers formerly regarded as charlatans or cranks are now becoming recognized (even registered) by the state, their knowledge now regarded as respectable by many, if not all. But it is also an aspect of an internal process of 'self-validation', an assertion of the cultural worth of the group's knowledge by its members for the benefit of other members, manifested in intragroup dialogue and debate. We could see, for example, Jeremy Sherr's interest in the periodic table as nothing more than part of a conscious strategy to prove the cultural worth of homoeopathic knowledge to those who are not convinced of it. The kind of discourse I have quoted here may in some cases be so motivated but it is probably more helpful to think of it in terms of (to take the same specific example) Jeremy Sherr finding that an idea he encounters in another body of knowledge with which he is familiar has applications in homoeopathy, and then seeking to share this with other homoeopaths. He has, after all, been inspired by his interest in the periodic table actually to conduct practical investigation of new remedies, and to circulate the results among the homoeopathic community. He does more than merely refer to the periodic table to justify his own ideas; he uses his knowledge of it to create further (homoeopathic) knowledge. Cultural legitimation is a diffuse process which operates within the profession as well as on its frontiers, though it is certainly also true that apologetics and professional rhetoric have a part to play in it.

A major trend in sociological thinking, however, has been to stress the fragmentation of knowledge in postmodernity, the lack of any overall system for the validation of knowledge now that science, let alone philosophy, can no longer fulfil that role. We have knowledges rather than knowledge, communities of knowers who participate in their own language games, with no metalanguage to connect them (Lyotard 1986: 41). Here is the view, as Geertz graphically and somewhat colloquially puts it, 'that things look more like flying apart than they do like coming together' (Geertz 1983: 216). At a more ethnographic level Geertz notes the 'metier-made mentalities' of different disciplines and communities of professionals or scholars and the 'deep dissimilarity of metier formed minds'. This leads him to ask whether and how it is possible for such inhabitants of specialized worlds ever to 'begin to find something circumstantial to each other again'. Geertz is perhaps more optimistic than most about the possibility of creating a vocabulary 'in which econometricians, epigraphers, cytochemists and iconographers can give a credible account of themselves to one another' (Geertz 1983: 161).

Not only may knowledge be fragmented into many local knowledges, but the anthropologist or sociologist him/herself may be so driven by the metanarrative of modernist rationalism (or some other overarching programme) that s/he over-emphasizes the systemic nature of the knowledge of specific professional or other communities; indeed exaggerates the extent to which they actually are communities or their knowledge unified. This is the import of a paper by the anthropologist David Parkin in the course of which he uses material from East Africa to demonstrate that the knowledge of healers who claim that their knowledge is in some sense 'Islamic' hardly constitutes a system (Parkin 1995). Nor indeed, in the context which Parkin describes, can one even separate 'religious' and 'medical' knowledge as distinct systems of thought. The religious and the medical are 'latticed' or 'intertwined' and the 'medical' certainly turns out to be a collection of ideas and practices which have little in the way of a unified system of verification. The healers

stay in business not on the basis of self-verifying faith, but through results which individual clients compare with each other and with those of other healers. It is healers' reputations which count, whatever we may regard as their empirical justification, and these require performative subtleties and novelties that defy the rigours of systems thinking. (Parkin 1995; 160–1)

Besides Parkin, Murray Last and Robert Pool – also working in African contexts – have strongly criticized the anthropologist's eagerness to identify 'systems' of medical knowledge (Last 1980; Pool 1994).

African medical pluralism has a different cultural genesis from that which we are seeing in countries like Britain today, but the critique can usefully be carried into the study of Western pluralism. From my own research experience I can say that it is certainly very easy to assume that because groups like the homoeopaths whom I have been discussing have been obliged to codify their knowledge (and to do this in a fairly public way in the interests of professional accountability), their knowledge is therefore necessarily highly systematized, that internal discontinuities and contradictions have been ironed out.

Turning from internal to external relationships, it does not follow, however, from the postmodernist proposition that the legitimation function of science has declined, that the resultant fragmented knowledges lack any other kind of mutual cultural connectedness at a practical level. We do not have to assume that they constitute groups based on highly local forms of knowledge with their own (again highly local) modes of verification which preclude integration or mutual communication. Performativity (both the kind noted locally by Parkin among clients of East African healers, and the kind noted more generally by Lyotard in modern/postmodern society), is certainly becoming an ever more important mode of legitimation; we can note the shift from the medical profession's insistence that complementary medicines *prove* the validity of their knowledge through laboratory trials and experiment to health authorities' insistence that complementary therapies *demonstrate* their practical efficacy and cost-effectiveness through appropriate forms of audit.

It is certainly useful to talk about knowledges rather than knowledge, but only so long as we recognize that there may be levels of interconnectedness, linkages which members of a professional group (and its critics) may variously wish to stress and develop, or downplay or deny (and some which may remain unacknowledged or implicit). In the case of the homoeopaths there has been an understandable desire on the part of some members of the professional community to stress the links between homoeopathic knowledge and science in any of a number of ways, understandable in terms of the prestige and power which science still holds and in terms of the insistence of others that their knowledge be shown to conform to science. Others have been indifferent to this mode of linkage or even opposed to it as a project. We can see this indifference as evidence of the decline in science's power to legitimate, but equally convincingly we can see it as the persistence of an earlier tradition of anti-rationalism, broader than but well represented in the Swedenborgianism of many nine-teenth-century homoeopaths (see Nicholls 1988: 259ff.).

The external linkages may, as we have seen, be of various types. It is seldom a case of straightforward overlap between bodies of knowledge; looking at the discourse of Society homoeopaths we can see linkages of highly diverse kinds – of contiguity, of analogy, of consistency, of situation, and so on. There is more than one way of locating your professional knowledge within a broader cultural landscape, though some may be more convincing than others. What these attempts at cultural situation tend to lack is a sense of hierarchy. The writers whom I have quoted have tried to link their homoeopathic knowledge to other forms of cultural knowledge, but not through the kind of intellectual devices which would allow one form of knowledge to legitimate or provide the rationale for another, let alone to subsume it. The links are always lateral and egalitarian, indeed, the spatial metaphor of the landscape[2] which I have just used suggests the two-dimensional horizontality of the map rather than the vertical extension of hierarchy. Where members of the Society of Homoeopaths have explored linkages with scientific knowledge it is always in a way that privileges the consistency between them as bodies of substantive knowledge rather than the conformity of homoeopathic knowledge to scientific method.

If homoeopaths are to be registered by the state and if they are to continue to have their services bought in by public health authorities, then in practice they are likely to be obliged to accept some practical domination by the medical profession, at least in the workplace. Already many training colleges recognized by the Society have felt it necessary to include some conventional medical scientific knowledge, particularly of anatomy, in their curricula. In as much as they aspire to work in the National Health Service they have to accept in practice the hierarchical division of labour/ knowledge enshrined in law and administration which situates other healing professions in relation to the medical profession itself. This hierarchy has become somewhat flattened as a result of recent changes, but it is nonetheless a hierarchy.

At the level of discourse about homoeopathic knowledge, however, we see a tendency to do away with hierarchies of knowledge altogether. The flatter the mutual disposition of knowledges, the better. Indeed we may recall Parkin's useful term 'latticing', developed in a somewhat different context, but referring to the lateral interweaving of different kinds of knowledge, often of diverse origins.

Whilst sociologists, anthropologists and other academicians may, with justification, perceive fragmentation to be the major condition of postmodern knowledge, a close examination of profession groups shows that in practice there are those who have not despaired of the project of a unified cultural knowledge, who yearn to go beyond mere 'performativity'. They may engage in a continual tinkering on the boundaries, a trafficking in knowledge between knowledge communities. In a situation where attempts to derive legitimation from labouring to 'prove' the conformity of homoeopathic knowledge to some branch of science or other will involve diminishing returns in relation to effort, they look to the construction of sideways linkages. The operative term here is 'constructive', for it is through such groups' efforts to situate themselves in a cultural landscape that a new cultural landscape might actually be fashioned.

Notes

1. I would like to record my gratitude to members and officers of the Society for the help they have provided. Much of this research was carried out as part of a project on Professionalization in Complementary Medicine, conducted with Sarah Cant and funded by the Economic and Social Research Council. Thanks are also due to Sarah herself for helpful comments on drafts of this paper and for much stimulus in the course of the project.
2. The metaphor of knowledge as landscape, or spatial territory, is embedded in English language usage. For a fuller discussion of the implications of this metaphor see Salmond (1982).

References

Andrews, M. (1994) 'The Periodic Table, Central Mind Symptoms, Chemical Properties and Uses'. *The Homoeopath* 54: 243.

Campbell, A. (1978) *The Two Faces of Homoeopathy*. London: Jill Norman.

Campbell, A. (1984) 'Is Homoeopathy Scientific? A Reassessment in the light of Karl Popper's Theory of Scientific Knowledge'. *British Homoeopathic Journal* 67: 77–85.

Cassam, A. (1994) 'Need Homoeopathy be a Science?'. *The Homoeopath* 54: 239–41.

Chera, L. (1994) 'Hecate Revisited'. *The Homoeopath* 55: 328–30.

Crompton, R. (1987) 'Gender, Status and Professionalism'. *Sociology* 21: 413–28.

Danciger, E. (1993) 'The Wounded Healer'. *The Homoeopath* 51: 130–2.

Fisher, P. (1981) 'Is Homoeopathy Scientific? A Reply to Anthony Campbell'. *British Homoeopathic Journal* 70: 152–8.

Geertz, C. (1983) *Local Knowledge. Further essays in Interpretive Anthropology.* NewYork: Basic Books.

Hahnemann, S. (1986) *Organon of Medicine.* New Delhi: B. Jain.

Holt, H. (1994) 'The Periodic Table'. *The Homoeopath* 54: 2766–7.

Last, M. (1980) 'The Importance of Knowing About Not Knowing'. *Social Science and Medicine* 15B: 387–92.

Lyotard, J. (1986) *The Postmodern Condition. A Report on Knowledge.* Manchester: Manchester University Press.

Maceoin, D. (1993) 'The Choice of Homoeopathic Models: The Patient's Dilemma'. *The Homoeopath* 51: 108–14.

Nicholls, P. (1988) *Homoeopathy and the Medical Profession.* London: Croom Helm.

Parkin, D. (1995) 'Latticed Knowledge. Eradication and Dispersal of the Unpalatable in Islam, Medicine and Anthropological Theory', in R. Fardon (ed.) *Counterworks; Managing the Diversity of Knowledge.* London: Routledge.

Pool, R. (1994) *Dialogue and the Intepretation of Illness.* Oxford: Berg.

Poitevin, B., Davenas, E. and Benveniste, J. (1988) 'In Vitro Immunological Degranulation of Human Basophils'. *British Journal of Clinical Pharmacology* 25: 439.

Rasool, J. (1994) 'Mind your Matter'. *The Homoeopath* 53: 205–9.

Robbins, B. (1993) *Secular Vocations. Intellectuals, Professionalism, Culture.* London: Verso.

Saks, M. (1995) *Professions and the Public Interest. Medical Power, Altruism and Alternative Medicine.* London: Routledge.

Salmond, A. (1982) 'Theoretical Landscapes. On a Cross-cultural Conception of Knowledge', in D. Parkin, (ed.) *Semantic Anthropology. Association of Social Anthropologists Monograph 22.* London: Academic Press.

Sherr, J. (1992) *The Homoeopathic Proving of Hydrogen.* Malvern: Jeremy Sherr.

Ullman, D. (1993) 'Understanding Nature to Learn Materia Medica'. *The Homoeopath* 13(1): 27–32.

Vannier, L. (1992) *Typology in Homoeopathy.* Beaconsfield: Beaconsfield Publishers.

Vithoulkas, G. (1980) *The Science of Homoeopathy.* New Delhi: B. Jain.

Wallis, R. and Morley, P. (eds) (1976) *Marginal Medicine.* London: Peter Owen.

Wansborough, C. J. (1995) 'Is Homoeopathy Becoming Dogmatic?'. *The Homoeopath* 57: 401–3.

Whitney, J. (1994) 'Views from the Conference; He-art and Sci-ence'. *Society of Homoeopaths Newsletter* December 1994, pp. 23–4.

Wright Hubbard, E. (1990) *Homoeopathy as Art and Science. Selected Writings.* Beaconsfield: Beaconsfield Publishers.

Final Observations

Sarah Cant and Ursula Sharma

This volume has served to extend a social scientific analysis to complementary medical knowledges. However, knowledge generation, as Giddens (1990) and Beck (1992) have theorized, produces both foreseen and unintended consequences which we should like to address in this concluding section.

It is clear that the expansion of complementary medicine could never have gone unnoticed by the medical profession, consumers, the state or indeed social scientists. Complementary therapies have been confronted by those bodies that have vested interests in the area of medical care (the orthodox medical profession), and those whose job it is to ensure the safety of the consumer and the public purse (the government). Such interested bodies have demanded that complementary medical groups prove that their knowledge is trustworthy and safe for others to sanction. Judgement of whether complementary medicine is legitimate has been based largely on conservative criteria, especially alignment to or distance from the established scientific paradigm. Complementary medical groups have seen their knowledge dismissed or accepted depending on the links to this, still powerful, metanarrative. Patients themselves may be less concerned with scientificity, not feeling that they need to understand the basis of the knowledge in order to benefit from it. We know that most patients make their decisions about which therapy and which practitioner to consult on the basis of the experiences of friends and family rather than on the basis of abstract judgements about legitimate knowledge.

However, complementary practitioners cannot survive on public demand alone and have had to engage with the scientific paradigm. At a practical level, of course, practitioners may encourage their patients' involvement and may dodge any 'legislative' function (see Introduction), preferring instead to interpret the information the patient offers, but to claim legitimacy and professional status they have had to stress their specialized expertise and, if only by implication, its distinctness from ordinary lay understanding. This demonstrates a contradiction in the nature of complementary medical knowledges, a contradiction that orthodox medicine may increasing have to face itself as it becomes more welcoming of the patients' perspective and more constrained by public demands for accountability and consumer involvement.

Complementary medical practitioners have been open to the interest shown by social scientists. Seeing themselves as a beleaguered group, the value of an advocate who can stress the satisfaction of patients and the vested interest of the medical profession must be appealing. Indeed our own research (Cant and Sharma 1994) was referred to by one group when making a case to the medical profession that it was involved in doing research about its own practice! Social scientific research can be seen as contributing to the campaign for acceptance and legitimacy.

But social scientific research may also have unforeseen consequences, possibly more problematic to the complementary professions. Bringing complementary medicines centre stage will also subject them to critical scrutiny and could raise questions in the public mind, just as the sociology of medicine has contributed to the public critique of orthodox medicine. The relativization of orthodox medical knowledge (seeing biomedicine as one among many cultural ways of knowing about the body) has been disturbing to some orthodox doctors; if complementary medicines find their knowledge subject to the same kind of cultural 'situation', may they not also be disturbed? For instance, the role of complementary medicines in the processes of medicalization has already been raised by Espen Braathen in this volume and will no doubt continue to be discussed. The material and professional interests at work in the social organization of complementary medical knowledge will be increasingly assessed, just as they have been in regard to orthodox medical knowledge. No longer will these groups be able to practise quietly away from the public gaze. Richenda Power's chapter illustrates the unease and dilemmas that such a shift in public accountability produces. Moreover, as we have seen, the changes that have been made to the knowledge bases have brought contradictions and confusion as well as rewards.

This collection has been an exciting enterprise. We, as editors, have learnt much about the role and practice of complementary medical knowledges. However, we have also been alerted to the dearth of information and to just how much more social scientific research needs to be done. It is important that the gender dimensions of complementary medicine be studied, that the role of complementary medical knowledges in ethnic communities be explored, that the experiences of the users be examined more thoroughly, that the changes in the relationship between the lay and the expert be charted and comprehended and that the tacit and uncodified knowledge of the practitioner in the consulting room and as gained in college be studied. Herein lies the challenge for future research.

What we hope that we have shown is that research on complementary medical knowledges can illuminate important debates about the role of knowledge in society. It is not (if it ever was) of purely marginal interest and curiosity value. We hope that we have been able to relate contemporary theory to the expanding volume of research being conducted in this field. The rise of complementary medical knowledge has practical implications for practitioners, patients and the medical division of labour, but also provides a contemporary case study through which to gain insight into how society might be changing more broadly.

References

Beck, U. (1992) Risk Society. London: Sage.
Cant, S. and Sharma, U. (1994) The Professionalisation of Complementary Medicine. Final Report to the ESRC.
Giddens, A. (1990) The Consequences of Modernity. Oxford: Polity.

Index

Bold numbers indicate pages on which there are illustrations.

Index by Auriol Griffith-Jones